THE 100 BEST WAYS TO STOP AGING AND STAY YOUNG

MOST METHODS TAKE 10 MINUTES OR LESS!

THE 100 BEST WAYS TO STOP AGING AND STAY YOUNG

SCIENTIFICALLY PROVEN STRATEGIES
FOR TAKING YEARS OFF YOUR BODY

JULIA MARANAN

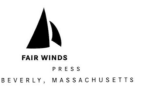

FAIR WINDS
PRESS
BEVERLY, MASSACHUSETTS

Text © 2011 Julia Maranan

First published in the USA in 2011 by
Fair Winds Press, a member of
Quayside Publishing Group
100 Cummings Center
Suite 406-L
Beverly, MA 01915-6101
www.fairwindspress.com

15 14 13 12 11   2 3 4 5

ISBN-13: 978-1-59233-449-0
ISBN-10: 1-59233-449-0

Library of Congress Cataloging-in-Publication Data available

Book design by Rachel Fitzgibbon, studio rkf
Photography by fotolia.com, istockphotos.com, and Thinkstock.com

Printed and bound in China

The information in this book is for educational purposes only. It is not intended to
replace the advice of a physician or medical practitioner. Please see your health-
care provider before beginning any new health program.

For Dan, who keeps me young.

I look forward to spending the rest of our years together.

Contents

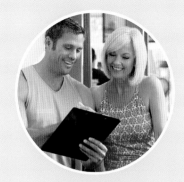
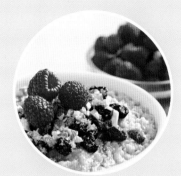
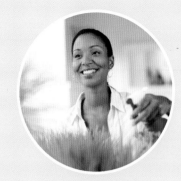

PART IV:

Turn Back the Clock on Your Bones and Joints

PART V:

Turn Back the Clock on Your Heart

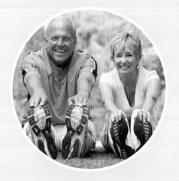
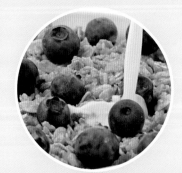
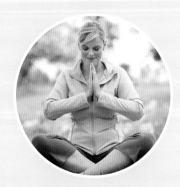

PART VI:

Turn Back the Clock on Your Immune System

PART VII:

Turn Back the Clock on Your Sex Life

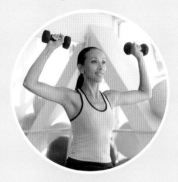
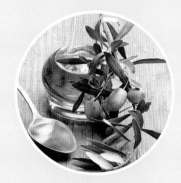
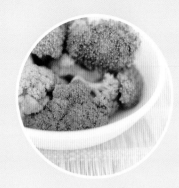

PART VIII:

Turn Back the Clock for More Energy

PART IX:

Important Dos and Don'ts to Slow the Aging Process

INTRODUCTION

Who doesn't want to live a longer, healthier, and happier life? My hope is that with this book, you can use these safe, effective, and scientifically proven tips to slow the aging process in a real and lasting way. The good news is that you don't have to overhaul your entire life—even making one or two changes can help you look and feel younger in just a few days or weeks. Once you get a few tips under your belt, add a few more to build on your success. It really is that easy, and whether you're thirty, sixty, or ninety, it's never too late (or too early!) to start.

Of course, on some days the healthier choices are easier to make than on others. But I often find that once I do one good thing for myself, I'm much more motivated to keep it up. It helps me to think of every day as filled with opportunities to take care of myself and ensure my good health for the long haul. The beauty of this book is that you have so many anti-aging options to choose from; if you don't feel like exercising one day, you can meet a friend for lunch instead and know that you're still keeping yourself young.

You might be surprised at all the ways you can slow the aging process. Even though I've been writing about health and nutrition for over a decade, in the course of writing this book I discovered many unexpected tips that turn back the clock. To be sure, your quickest path to anti-aging is adopting healthy habits such as eating more fruits and vegetables and exercising. But volunteering, cultivating an optimistic outlook, and forgiveness also play a big part. And did you know lifestyle changes like cutting back on refined carbs are twice as effective at preventing diabetes as medications?

Inexpensive and available to everyone, lifestyle changes such as these carry virtually no risk of side effects, and in many cases they're actually more effective than drugs, surgery, or other medical interventions. They are also, by far, the least expensive ways to maintain or restore good health. That translates into less time in the doctor's office, fewer medications, lower medical bills, and the good health and energy to keep doing the things you love for decades to come. If you've picked up this book, I imagine that's what you're hoping for as well. So start reading and begin turning back the clock today. Best wishes for a long, healthy, and happy life.

—*Julia Maranan*

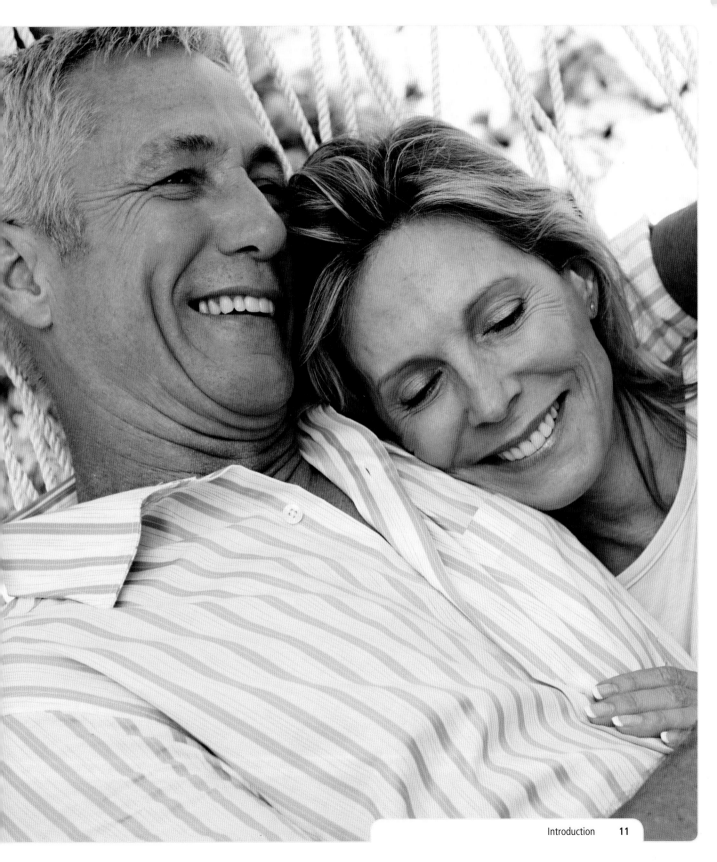

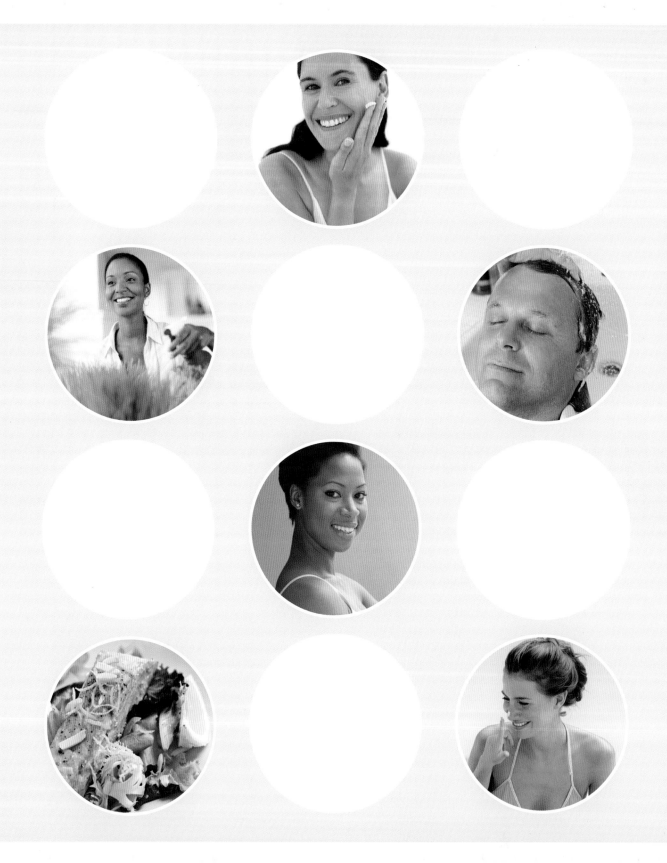

PART I

Turn Back the Clock on Your Face

Use Hyaluronic Acid to Fight Age-Related Wrinkles

As you get older, your skin undergoes changes at every level. The top layer (the epidermis) thins and loses protective fatty substances called lipids, making skin drier and less able to fight off infection. Arid climates or the dry air in winter can aggravate parched skin even more. Dry skin can feel tight and uncomfortable, accentuate wrinkles, and look flaky and ashy. Also as you age, the inner layer (the dermis)—the collagen and elastic tissues that keep your skin firm and plump—begins to break down, leading to wrinkles. These changes mean your skin doesn't bounce back from injury as quickly.

Enter moisturizers, which can help calm itchiness and irritation, plump and smooth skin, and restore a youthful, dewy look. One hydrating hero is hyaluronic acid (aka sodium hyaluronate), which is naturally found in skin. A 2004 study in *Skin Pharmacology and Physiology* noted that hyaluronic acid boosts production of cells that make and secrete collagen, at the same time shoring up skin's structure.

Hyaluronic acid moisturizes skin from the inside, increases elasticity, calms inflammation, and scavenges skin-damaging free radicals. As you get older, you produce less hyaluronic acid, which can lead to dry skin and wrinkles. The good news? Applying it topically seems to restore some of those benefits, plumping and firming skin almost immediately. It can hold up to one thousand times its weight in water and helps attract and bind moisture to your skin, even in concentrations as low as 1 percent (although you may see more noticeable results with higher concentrations). It's easily absorbed and may also help other skin-saving ingredients penetrate the skin better, making combination products more effective.

You can find topical hyaluronic acid in moisturizers at all price points (starting at under $10) in serums, creams, gels, and so on, often alongside other anti-aging ingredients to give you multiple benefits in one bottle.

Injectable Hyaluronic Acid Fills in Wrinkles That Come with Age

Researchers at Cambridge University in England note that injectable hyaluronic acid works best for deep wrinkles caused by sun damage, creases around the nose and mouth, and adding volume to hollowed cheeks and thin lips (areas that Botox, which works best on forehead wrinkles, can't help). Manufacturers chemically modify it so that skin doesn't absorb it as quickly, which means results can last up to six

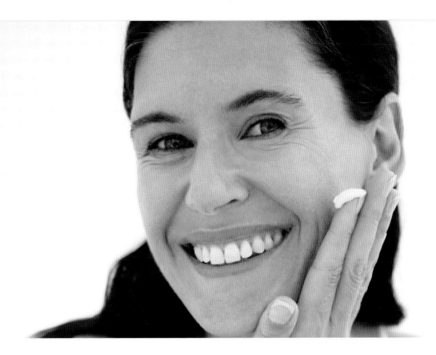

months. Using it repeatedly in the same area may lead to a longer-lasting result, possibly by stimulating new collagen production. Injectable hyaluronic acid is available in heavier and lighter gels with different molecule sizes, which translates to more flexibility for where on your face you can use it. Another plus is that most people tolerate it well; irritation and allergic reactions are rare.

Good Skin Care Habits Prolong a Youthful Glow

All the potions and anti-agers in the world can't undo the damage from poor skin care habits. Even if you have a good regimen in place, as you get older your routine might need some tweaks. If your skin is still dry even though you use a moisturizer with hyaluronic acid, start washing your face only at night. Make sure you use a mild, soap-free cleanser (one study rated Dove, Aveeno,

and Purpose as the least irritating) and lukewarm water to avoid stripping skin of its natural oils. In the morning, simply wet your skin and pat it dry with a towel. The other two crucial components to younger-looking skin? Don't skimp on sunscreen (▶**2**) and stop smoking (▶**93**).

The Takeaway: Moisturizing Musts

Apply a moisturizer with hyaluronic acid right after you wash your face to lock in moisture; men should use moisturizer after shaving.

If you have sensitive skin, look for fragrance-free formulas rather than unscented, which just use chemicals to cover up smells.

If you're acne-prone (yes, even adults can get pimples!), look for an oil-free moisturizer labeled noncomedogenic and non-acnegenic to banish breakouts.

2

Shield Yourself from the Aging Effects of the Sun

By some estimates, sun exposure accounts for nearly 90 percent of age-related damage to often-exposed areas such as the face, the back of the neck and "V" of the neckline, the arms, and the backs of the hands. Why, exactly, does the sun pose such a problem? Ultraviolet radiation falls into three wavelengths, but only two reach the earth: ultraviolet A (UVA) and ultraviolet B (UVB). UVA rays are responsible for long-term photoaging, while UVBs are the culprit behind sunburn. Both types create free radicals that damage healthy skin cells and make it harder for skin to heal, and both play a role in skin cancer. Ultraviolet radiation breaks down elastin and speeds up collagen loss, leading to wrinkles. It can also make your skin thicker in some areas and thinner in others, affecting skin tone and texture. You can chalk up brown spots and spider veins to sun damage as well. And while fair-skinned people tend to have more visible signs of photoaging than those with dark skin, UV rays penetrate deeply, damaging skin and increasing the risk of skin cancer regardless of your skin color.

Sunscreen Protects and Even Heals Sun-Damaged Skin

Slathering on sunscreen is a smart strategy for both preventing and undoing sun damage. A *New England Journal of Medicine* study looked at nearly six hundred people over the age of forty and found that using SPF 17 every day not only shielded them from harmful rays, it actually allowed sun-damaged skin to heal as well. To get the most benefit from sunscreen, apply a broad-spectrum formula of at least SPF 15 (if you have fair skin or burn easily, opt for SPF 30) half an hour before heading outdoors—even on cloudy days. Reapply every two hours, especially if you're sweating, wet, or have dried or rubbed your skin with a towel.

Selecting a Sunscreen to Keep Your Skin Young

A 2009 study found that adding antioxidants like vitamins C and E and epigallocatechin-3-gallate (EGCG) in green tea to a broad-spectrum sunscreen makes it even more effective in preventing sun damage. Since no sunscreen can block all UV rays, some radiation does get through to skin and creates free radicals. The antioxidants quench free radicals before they age your skin. Look for products with sun protection and antioxidants in one bottle.

There are two types of sunscreens: physical and chemical. Physical sunscreens contain ingredients such as zinc oxide and titanium dioxide that scatter or reflect UVA and UVB

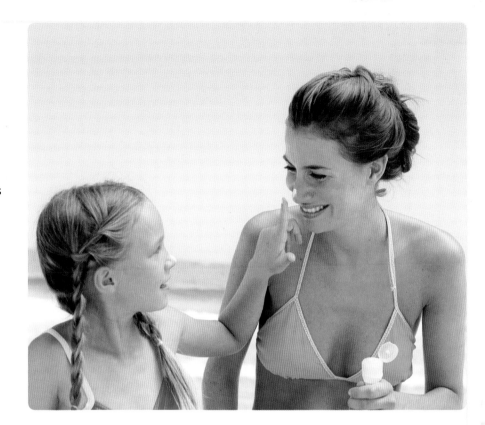

rays so they can't penetrate the skin. Remember lifeguards with those white stripes down their noses? They were using physical sunscreens. Thankfully, recent formulations are better able to blend in with your skin and are less noticeable. Physical sunscreens are popular picks for people with sensitive skin or rosacea.

Chemical sunscreens usually rely on one or more active ingredients—such as avobenzone (Parsol 1789), oxybenzone, or newcomer mexoryl (Anthelios SX)—to absorb UVA and UVB rays before they can damage skin. If you choose a chemical sunscreen, make sure it's broad spectrum to protect against both UVA and UVB rays.

Clinically Proven Damage Control for Older Skin

To repair sun-damaged skin, most dermatologists agree that prescription-only tretinoin, or Retin-A, is the top treatment. In a 2009 study, French researchers found that with nine months of regular application, a 0.1 percent retinol treatment improved under-eye wrinkles, fine lines, and skin tone. Research shows that 0.05 percent Retin-A cream helps heal mild to moderate photodamage as well. Retin-A protects against collagen breakdown and actually repairs collagen and elastic fibers, restoring collagen production by about 80 percent over ten to twelve months of daily use, according to a *New England Journal of Medicine* study. It

also improves wrinkles and skin texture and color. Retin-A can cause irritation and redness, so talk to your doctor if you experience these side effects. It also increases your sensitivity to sunlight, so be superdiligent about wearing sunscreen while you use it. Over-the-counter products with retinols offer more subtle benefits.

Alpha hydroxy acids, vitamin C, and peptides are worthy additions to your skin-repair arsenal as well (▶7).

3

Eat Omega-3s for Younger-Looking Skin

Skin is the body's largest living organ, and it needs top-notch nourishment to function and look its best. While a healthy diet filled with fruits and vegetables, whole grains, lean protein, and good fats (▶13) will work wonders for your appearance, a few skin superstars are worth working into your diet for their anti-aging benefits.

Omega-3 and Omega-6 Fatty Acids Protect against Skin Aging

You've probably heard about the benefits of omega-3s for heart health (▶58) and the brain (▶25). But mounting research shows that they, along with omega-6s, are also critical for skin health and can fight signs of aging. These essential fatty acids calm inflammation and irritation caused by free radicals. They keep cell membranes fluid and flexible and normalize oil production by creating protective lipids

(fatty substances) in your skin's topmost layer—especially helpful as your skin gets drier with age, and since dry skin makes wrinkles more noticeable (▶1). Omega-3s and omega-6s also defend against cell damage and assist in repair, keeping skin resilient. A 2006 review of studies concluded that consuming omega-3s can actually protect skin from sun damage as well.

Omega-3s and omega-6s are called essential fatty acids because our bodies can't make them, so we have to get them through diet. Omega-6s are abundant in foods like eggs, vegetable oils, poultry, and grains, and most people consume more than enough. The trick is getting enough omega-3s. Omega-3s are a group of several nutrients, including eicosapentaenoic acid (EPA) and docosahexaenoic acid (DHA). Fatty, cold-water fish like wild salmon, lake

trout, albacore tuna, herring, anchovies, and sardines are among the best sources. Surprisingly, grass-fed beef also offers a respectable amount. Omega-3-fortified eggs and other fortified foods are another option. Walnuts, ground flaxseed, and soy foods like tofu provide another omega-3 known as alpha-linolenic acid (ALA), which the body can use to make EPA and DHA. Broccoli, cabbage, and other leafy greens also supply small amounts of ALA.

Add Age-Fighting Antioxidants

Like omega-3s and omega-6s, antioxidant vitamins A, C, and E fight free radicals that can damage skin and lead to wrinkles and even skin cancer. Topical antioxidants get a lot of press (▶7), but your primary goal should be to get enough through diet. Brightly colored fruits and vegetables, such as avocados, broccoli, carrots, kiwis, nuts

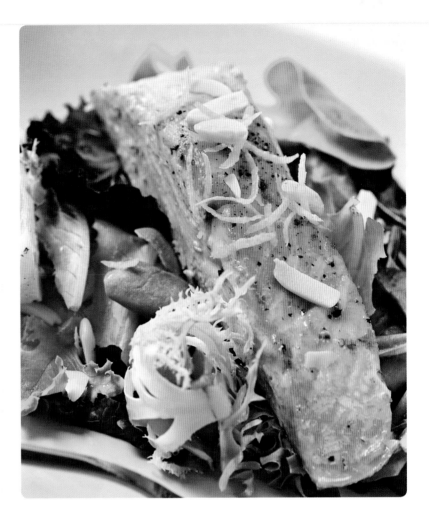

The Takeaway: Healthy Fats for Healthy Skin

Eating two 3- to 4-ounce servings of oily fish a week is the easiest way to get enough omega-3s.

If your diet falls short, talk to your doctor about taking a fish oil supplement (▶58) that contains 500 milligrams or more of EPA and DHA or one made from algae that has 400 to 600 milligrams of DHA.

and seeds, oranges, red and green peppers, spinach, and strawberries are super sources. It can be tough to get enough vitamin E from foods, but you should talk to your doctor if you're thinking about supplementing, since vitamin E can act as a blood thinner, and high levels may interfere with cholesterol-lowering drugs. If you choose to supplement with vitamin E, take 400 IU of mixed natural tocopherols daily (d-alpha tocopherol is the natural form; avoid synthetic dl-alpha tocopherol).

Include Minerals in Your Anti-Aging Diet

A 2009 study noted that people with high levels of selenium in their blood reduced their risk of skin cancer by about 60 percent. Its antioxidant action helps prevent premature skin aging, and it encourages vitamin E absorption as well. Good sources include brown rice, seafood, garlic, eggs, and Brazil nuts.

Another multitasker, zinc, protects your skin from sun damage and works with vitamin C to make collagen. A zinc

deficiency can trigger breakouts, lead to hair loss, and cause rough skin or rashes. Food sources include oysters, legumes (such as beans and peas), red meat, pecans, and pumpkin seeds. If you don't eat many animal foods, you might want to supplement, but the National Institutes of Health Office of Dietary Supplements recommends getting no more than 40 milligrams per day.

4 Use Psychodermatology to Keep Older Skin Supple

Your eyes may be the window to your soul, but your skin is a pretty good indicator of your emotional health. In fact, experts are realizing that the connection between emotions and skin is so strong that they've coined a term for this growing field: psychodermatology. Dermatologists have long recognized that stress can make your skin more sensitive and worsen conditions such as acne, eczema, and rosacea, but research reveals that it can also add years to your appearance. For example, stress dehydrates skin, and a 2009 study in the *Journal of Biomechanics* found that reducing moisture in the skin's top layer by 11 percent produces wrinkles that are 25 to 85 percent larger. Stress also breaks down skin-firming collagen and slows your body's ability to make more collagen. Additionally, stress can increase skin inflammation, leading to

itchiness, flushing, and uneven skin tone. If that weren't bad enough, in addition to the direct effects of stress on your skin, anxiety often causes people to neglect good skin-care habits or abuse their skin by rubbing, pulling, or picking at it. But before you resort to hiding your head under a paper bag, there are plenty of ways you can tame tension (▶ **18, 56, 61**) and stop its aging effects on your skin. Feeling good about your skin's appearance may reduce stress and anxiety in other parts of your life as well. Here are some stress-busting, skin-saving tips.

Take a Deep Breath to Revive Aging Skin

When people get worked up, their breathing often gets shallower. Some people even hold their breath without realizing it, thanks to muscle tension throughout the body. Breathing deeply not only helps you unwind, but it allows

you to take in more oxygen, which nourishes and refreshes the skin. Even better, that extra oxygen also signals skin to produce collagen, plumping your skin and helping to prevent wrinkles.

Besides making an effort to breathe normally throughout the day, you might want to try this simple breathing technique from Andrew Weil, M.D., an expert in natural healing and healthy aging, to relax and recharge whenever you need a lift. First, place the tip of your tongue just behind your upper front teeth (keep it there throughout the exercise). Exhale completely through your mouth, making a whooshing sound. Inhale quietly through your nose while you count to four. Hold your breath for seven counts, then exhale through your mouth (making the whoosh sound again) for a count of eight. Repeat the cycle four times. Kiss those worry lines goodbye!

Exercise to Erase Stress and Keep Skin Young

A 2007 study in *Biological Research for Nursing* looked at adults over age sixty and noted that thirty minutes of walking at 60 percent of their maximum heart rate (considered moderate exercise) significantly lowered stress and improved mood after ten weeks. In addition, a 2009 study in the *European Journal of Applied Physiology* measured circulation to the skin in postmenopausal women after they had exercised for twenty-four, thirty-six, and forty-eight weeks and found that it continued to improve the longer the women had been exercising.

Exercise is perhaps the best stress reliever there is (even as little as ten minutes of movement can stop stress in its tracks, which is a pretty remarkable return on investment), and it offers both short- and long-term benefits. For immediate impact, exercise helps burn off extra energy when tension has you tied in knots, and it boosts circulation to bring nutrients to the skin, remove toxins, and improve skin tone. In the long run, it helps keep your stress hormones balanced, allowing you to stay calm even in the face of chronic chaos. In 2008, University of Colorado researchers performed a series of animal studies showing that regular exercise modifies the way the body responds to the stress hormone cortisol, ultimately reducing the amount the body and brain are exposed to. Reducing your exposure to cortisol could translate to keeping skin better hydrated, boosting collagen production, and calming inflammation.

The Takeaway: Relieve Stressed Skin

Feeling anxious? Set a reminder on your Outlook calendar or your phone to remind you to breathe deeply or do breathing exercises throughout the day.

To get the best stress-busting effects of exercise, you should enjoy it, so how you get moving—a brisk walk or run, lifting weights, yoga or stretching, dancing, or hitting a punching bag—is up to you.

5

Stop Squinting to Preserve Firmness

Repetitive facial movements, like squinting or frowning, form grooves beneath the skin's surface every time the facial muscles contract. That repeated wear and tear causes changes in the connective tissue and breaks down the extracellular matrix, skin's support structure. As you age, your skin can't snap back into place as easily, and over time those grooves become wrinkles, according to the American Academy of Dermatology. This accounts for the astronomic rise in popularity of botulinum toxin (Botox), which paralyzes the small muscles used to create fixed expression lines (▶II). Botox does carry risks, however, and you can safely make simple lifestyle changes to reduce your likelihood of getting these types of wrinkles (and possibly even minimize existing ones).

Sleep Beautifully to Reduce Age Lines

The American Academy of Dermatology notes that people who sleep on their sides or stomach tend to smoosh their faces into their pillows. If you sleep in the same position every night, sleep lines can form along the chin and cheeks (if you're a side sleeper) or the forehead (if you sleep facedown). As your skin loses elasticity with age, the lines stick around even when you're not resting your head on a pillow. The answer? Sleep on your back if you can, or at least vary your sleeping position from day to day. The jury is still out on new pillowcases and bedding that are infused with copper, aloe, and other substances that claim to confer beauty benefits while you sleep. But if you try changing your sleeping position and still find yourself with your face crumpled against your pillow in the morning, a satin pillowcase is an inexpensive option to try. The smooth fabric may allow your skin to lay flat when pressed against it. And even if it doesn't help solve your sleep lines, it's a luxurious touch that you can enjoy for other reasons.

You may have heard about Hollywood stars using adhesive strips called Frownies to prevent them from making wrinkle-forming facial expressions while they sleep. Despite positive customer testimonials, in a 2009 study in the *Archives of Facial Plastic Surgery*, plastic surgeons looked at photos of subjects before and after four weeks of using Frownies. The surgeons, who were not told which were the before and which were the after photos, found no change in wrinkles. Still, the subjects in the study did think they saw slight improvement. If you tend to frown in your sleep, Frownies are a relatively inexpensive experiment. But you might also get the same benefit by using a (basically free) strip of tape.

Find Flattering Frames to Keep Crow's Feet at Bay

Crow's feet—wrinkles around the outside corner of your eyes—are largely due to squinting. Get in the habit of wearing sunglasses (with 100 percent UV protection to shield eyes and the surrounding delicate skin from sun damage) outdoors, even in winter. In fact, sunlight reflecting off snow can be even brighter than the summer sun.

You should also get an eye exam to see if you need glasses or if your prescription has changed. According to the Vision Council of America, 172.3 million American adults wear a form of vision correction, either glasses or contacts. And the older you get, the more likely you'll need prescription eyewear, even if you've had excellent vision all your life. Getting the correct prescription—and wearing it religiously—ensures that you won't need to squint to read the fine print.

Relax Your Face to Stave Off Wrinkles

If you furrow your brow, purse your lips, or frown when you're concentrating, worried, or displeased, mom was right: Your face will freeze like that. Well, not exactly, but these repetitive movements can lead to wrinkling. Try to be mindful of making pronounced facial expressions, and if you catch yourself doing it, relax your facial muscles into a more neutral and restful position.

Also, skip exercising—for your face, that is. Programs that promise to tone your facial muscles through repetitive motions or resistance actually create wrinkles. Because skin loses elasticity as it ages, every time you perform a repetitive facial motion your skin doesn't bounce back to its wrinkle-free state as easily. Over time, these exercises essentially carve wrinkles into your skin. Not quite what you had intended, right?

The Takeaway: Wrinkle Prevention

Wear sunglasses every day.

Get an eye exam to be sure your prescription is correct.

Keep your facial expressions in neutral.

6

Use More than Moisturizer to Heal Mature Skin

If you've noticed your skin getting drier with age, you're not alone. Over time, the outermost layer of your epidermis (the stratum corneum) loses lipids, the fatty substances that protect and keep your skin moist. And it's not limited to the skin on your face: You might notice dry, itchy, easily irritated skin all over your body, especially in winter. Besides being uncomfortable, dry skin can make wrinkles more noticeable and lead to flaky, ashy skin—quite the opposite of the dewy complexion of your youth.

Humidify and Hydrate to Plump Wrinkled Skin

Whether it's due to an arid climate or indoor heating, lack of moisture in the air can make a big difference in how dry your skin feels. A 2007 study in the *Journal of Biomedical Optics* found that increasing the relative humidity of the air causes skin to plump up, potentially diminishing wrinkles. To combat dry air, use a humidifier in your bedroom at night. If you have radiators, you can also place a tray of water on top—the heat will cause the water to evaporate and add moisture back into the air. Keeping well-watered houseplants nearby will also raise humidity. An inexpensive hygrometer, available at hardware stores or online, can track humidity levels; aim for 50 percent humidity (and no less than 30 percent, the amount at which skin starts to feel uncomfortably dry).

Although only a small percentage of the water you consume ends up reaching your skin, there's no denying the importance of staying hydrated. Experts are divided on how much water you need to consume daily, and it varies according to your health, climate, and activity level. But as a general recommendation, the Institute of Medicine suggests that men consume roughly thirteen cups (about 3 L) and women consume nine cups (about 2.2 L) of total beverages a day. Notice that they didn't just say "water." That means that drinks such as milk, tea, and juice, plus foods with high water content such as grapes, tomatoes, and melon, all count toward your total. And there's extra good news for those who enjoy hot beverages to take the chill off: A 2006 study in the *Journal of Nutrition* found that women who drank cocoa with high levels of flavanols (antioxidant compounds) had better-hydrated and smoother skin than women who drank low-flavanol cocoa. Look for varieties made with chocolate containing at least 60 percent cocoa to get a similar benefit. Marshmallows are optional.

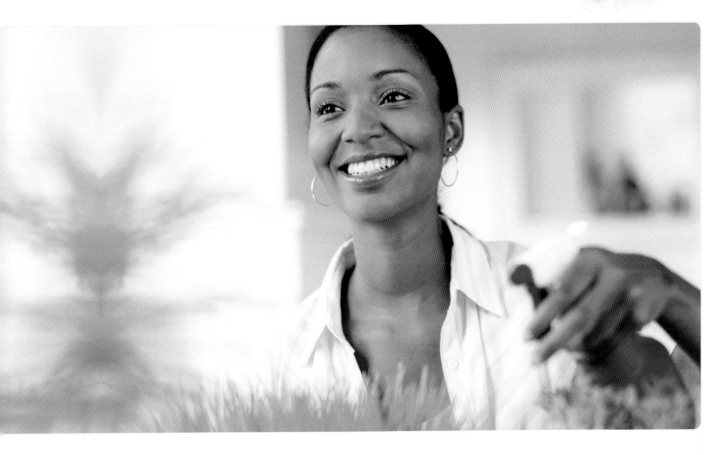

Water Can Actually Dry Out Aging Skin

Surprisingly, water isn't always good for keeping skin moist. Long, hot showers may do wonders for your psyche, but they wreak havoc with your skin. Hot water strips natural oils more quickly, so use warm, not hot, water for showers and baths. And limit yourself to five to ten minutes in the water—any longer than that is actually dehydrating, according to the American Academy of Dermatology.

Steer clear of deodorant, antibacterial, or strongly scented soaps, which are too harsh, and avoid alcohol-based toners and cleansers. Dry skin is often more sensitive, so don't derail your anti-aging efforts by exfoliating too much or too harshly with peels or scrubbing. Use milder treatments (or use them less frequently) until after you've tried these tips and your skin is better hydrated and less sensitive.

As water evaporates from the surface of your skin, it actually pulls moisture out of the skin's top layer, exacerbating dryness. So the best time to moisturize is right after you shower or wash your face, while your skin is still slightly damp. Creams work best for sealing in moisture; rely on rich formulas with hyaluronic acid (▶I), shea butter, ceramides, stearic acid, or glycerin. For severely dry skin, try a moisturizer that contains urea or lactic acid—the American Academy of Dermatology notes that they help the skin hold water if used regularly. For cracked skin, Aquaphor is the dermatologist's treatment of choice.

The Takeaway: Hydrate Skin

Humidify your home.

Drink plenty of water.

Wash with warm, not hot, water.

7

Repair Aging Skin at Night

You already know that wearing sunscreen during the day is your first defense against aging skin (▶2). Many dermatologists suggest saving anti-aging creams to use at night, since sunlight can inactivate some of the ingredients or cause irritation—plus, they don't have to compete with sunscreen and makeup to penetrate your skin.

Peptides Promise to Reduce Signs of Aging

When collagen breaks down, it forms short chains of amino acids called peptides that spur skin to repair itself. Applying peptides topically may trick your skin into thinking it needs to make more collagen. Moreover, because it's easy to modify the molecules to help them cross the skin barrier more effectively, peptide formulations can carry other helpful ingredients to the skin and decrease toxicity, according

to a 2009 study in the *Journal of Cosmetic Dermatology*.

Peptide treatments are relatively new to the market—in fact, much of the existing research focuses on peptides as wound-healing agents or as a way to deliver other ingredients to the skin—but dermatologists quickly saw their potential for helping reduce signs of aging. For instance, peptides typically bind water and, therefore, help hydrate skin, says Mary Lupo, M.D., dermatologist and professor at Tulane Medical School. That especially benefits aging skin, since skin gets drier as you mature and dry skin accentuates wrinkles.

There are three main types of peptides with anti-aging benefits. Signal peptides increase collagen production and reduce fine lines. Carrier peptides deliver copper to the skin, triggering a

wound-healing response that boosts collagen and may improve skin tone and hyperpigmentation, as well as diminish fine lines. Neurotransmitter-inhibiting peptides may actually decrease muscle movement, leading to a mild Botox-like effect. Lab studies are encouraging, but it remains to be seen if these kinds of peptides can actually penetrate deep enough to reach the nerve-muscle connection in humans.

Within these three main categories, individual peptides are proprietary and licensed to cosmetics companies, notes Lupo. Many different peptides are available in a variety of products, but you'll frequently see (signal) pentapeptides (found in StriVectin at $50 to $100 a pop, or Olay's Regenerist line, in the $20 range) and copper peptides (such as Neova, in the $75 range, or Neutrogena's Visibly Firm line

Introduce one new product at a time to your skin-care regimen to see how your skin reacts. Allow six to twelve weeks to see results. Follow package directions to avoid irritation; more does not always mean better!

Try new peptides as well as trusted alpha hydroxy acid (AHA) products and formulations that include antioxidant vitamins C, E, and A.

for under $30) on labels. Experts predict combination products with multiple types will be next to hit shelves.

Tried and True Topicals for Tired Skin

In the past few years, peptides have stolen the skin-care spotlight, but don't dismiss ingredients that have been around longer; many have strong evidence supporting their effectiveness. These anti-agers have more research behind them, and dermatologists regularly recommend them to renew aging skin.

Alpha hydroxy acids can boost collagen and elastic fibers and hydrate skin if used regularly. Effective exfoliators, they also slough off dead skin cells that make skin dull and reduce the appearance of fine wrinkles. When shopping for AHAs, such as lactic and glycolic acids, which

have been studied the most for safety and effectiveness, stick to over-the-counter concentrations of 10 percent or less and a pH of at least 3.5. Alpha Hydrox ($10 range), DDF ($35 to $50), and Peter Thomas Roth ($35 and up) are all good picks. AHAs make your skin more sun sensitive, so be diligent about wearing sunscreen and avoiding sun exposure while using them.

Solid research, including a 2006 review of studies in *Dermatologic Surgery*, confirms vitamin C's benefits for skin, including boosting collagen production, protecting against sun damage, lightening dark skin spots, and calming inflammation. L-ascorbic acid seems to be the most effective form; ideally, a product will contain at least a 10 percent concentration. Check out certain Cellex-C products ($100 to $150) and La Roche-Posay's Active C line ($35 to $50).

Vitamin C degrades quickly when exposed to light and air, so look for products in single-use or opaque packaging. Use within ninety days of opening, and consider storing it in the refrigerator.

Other topical antioxidants, such as green tea, coenzyme Q10, and vitamin E, also get the dermatologist seal of approval for their ability to quench free radicals.

Prescription-strength retinoids, such as Retin-A (tretinoin), are dermatologists' first choice for repairing sun damage (▶2). Milder over-the-counter formulas of these vitamin A derivatives, called retinols, offer some anti-aging benefits as well. Try certain Philosophy products ($40 to $60), the ROC line ($10 to $45), and the Neutrogena Ageless Intensives line ($20). They can irritate skin, so start with a small amount every other day and build up to daily application.

8

Use Treatments at Home to Take Years Off

Anti-aging treatments that once were offered only in the dermatologist's office are now increasingly available at home. Microdermabrasion kits and chemical peels are two of the most popular. Both treatments work by exfoliating, which brings several benefits. First, mature skin is usually drier, and dead cells don't slough off as easily, which translates to fine lines, rougher texture, and uneven skin tone. Exfoliation removes those cells and reveals younger, fresher skin underneath. Those new skin cells are better able to hold on to moisture, and they allow other anti-aging ingredients to penetrate better and work more effectively.

Because at-home treatments contain a lower concentration of active ingredients, do-it-yourself results can't match those from the doctor's office, but using them regularly can produce noticeable results at a fraction of the cost. And the American Academy of Dermatology notes that at-home treatments "can be safe when they have been thoroughly tested for this type of self-use"—as long as you follow the package directions. Here's what you need to know if you'd like to try them on your own.

Renew Mature Skin with Microdermabrasion

For an in-office microdermabrasion treatment, a dermatologist uses a wand to spray the skin with small crystals, such as aluminum oxide, providing deep exfoliation. This helps diminish fine lines and brown spots, and improves skin tone and texture. Skin fully recovers within twenty-four hours, and many patients notice some improvement right away, although you'll likely need multiple sessions spread over several weeks for clearly visible results. At-home kits use similar technology, but the exfoliation isn't as deep. Still, regular microdermabrasion treatments enhance skin cell turnover and will leave you with softer, smoother skin and fewer fine lines. The most basic products are simply grainy scrubs that you rub on your face with your fingertips.

A 2009 study in the *Journal of Dermatological Treatment* found that applying topical antioxidants immediately after professional microdermabrasion increased the number of fibroblasts, cells that produce collagen. Using an antioxidant-rich moisturizer or serum (such as Juice Beauty Antioxidant Serum [$45] or Neutrogena Anti-Oxidant Age Reverse moisturizers [$20]) after at-home microdermabrasion may offer similar benefits. And of course, be sure to protect your new, softer skin with sunscreen during the day (▶2).

Reveal Younger Skin with Chemical Peels

Mild chemical peels usually rely on alpha hydroxy acids (AHAs) like lactic acid, glycolic acid, or citric acid to exfoliate skin and encourage younger, healthier skin to develop. Unlike microdermabrasion, which physically removes dead skin cells from the skin's top layer, chemical peels dissolve the "glue" that holds cells together so they can slough off. The result is softer, brighter skin with less-noticeable signs of sun damage, such as fine lines, wrinkles, and age spots. At-home peels use lower concentrations of the acids—typically between 5 and 15 percent, compared to 30 percent for an in-office glycolic acid peel, for example. That means results aren't as dramatic, but with regular use the less-potent treatments are still effective.

All the same, you are dealing with acids in concentrations high enough to cause irritation and other problems with overuse, so stick to well-known brands (such as Olay or other common drugstore brands, or those found in specialty stores like Ulta or Sephora, which likely have better safety track records) and always follow the directions. Chemical peels work best to reverse the effects of sun damage when they're used along with other anti-aging treatments, noted a study in the 2008 issue of *Clinics in Dermatology*. Common combinations include microdermabrasion, Retin-A, and antioxidants (▶2, 7). To be safe, check with your dermatologist before using an at-home peel in case any of the ingredients interact with anti-agers you're already using. And as always, you'll need to be religious about using sunscreen so you don't undo all your results.

The Takeaway: Exfoliate Skin

For microdermabrasion products, look for small, smooth particles, since large or rough ones can tear and damage skin.

Another option is handheld devices with foam pads or brushes, which you use to massage creams with crystals or other exfoliating particles evenly into the skin.

People with sensitive skin might prefer peels because they offer chemical exfoliation, which is gentler than manual exfoliation from microdermabrasion.

9

Supercharge Your Smile to Look Younger

Your skin is not the only feature to show your age—your smile can give you away too. As you get older, the enamel on your teeth wears away, which can result in chips, yellowing, and stains. Your gums naturally start to recede as well. Around age thirty-five, the elastic tissues around your mouth begin to break down, and the fat that gives volume and plumpness slowly disappears, leading to thinner, flatter lips. You may also notice that the corners of your mouth are starting to droop, and lip lines have begun to form (especially in smokers). Your dentist and dermatologist have a few tricks up their sleeves if you'd like to pursue professional treatments, but inexpensive lifestyle changes and products can also address many of these telltale signs.

Try a Dental Face-Lift to Erase Years from Your Look

A 2010 study in *Plastic and Reconstructive Surgery* found that the bones in the jaw also lose volume as you age; the researchers concluded that the combination of soft tissue changes and having less bony support causes cheeks to appear hollow and skin to sag, and this can worsen wrinkles. A recent trend to combat those signs of aging is a procedure often called a smile lift or dental face-lift. It usually involves using veneers, crowns, or other orthodontic devices to change the shape of your teeth, potentially lifting your lips, broadening your smile, and reducing fine lines. If your dentist doesn't have experience with this kind of anti-aging dentistry, check with the American Academy of Cosmetic Dentistry to find a cosmetic dentist in your area. It can be expensive, since each procedure

is highly personalized (a few veneers might cost a few hundred dollars, for example, but a whole mouthful of veneers plus orthodontic devices and other procedures can run into the five-figure range), but the results can be dramatic.

If you're looking for less costly ways to restore your smile, you might also try an injectable filler from your dermatologist. Unlike Botox, which paralyzes muscles to keep them from creating wrinkles, these fillers—usually hyaluronic acid (▶I), collagen, or the body's own fat—fill in wrinkles and deeper folds, help restore loss of volume, and soften the contours of the face (▶II). Cost varies according to the filler you choose, but the average cost was around $500 in 2008, according to the American Society of Plastic Surgeons. Although soft tissue fillers are generally considered safe,

The Takeaway: Smile Enhancers

Berry-colored lipstick and over-the-counter tooth-whitening strips are low-cost brighteners.

Injectable fillers and dental-office whitening are midrange options.

A dental lift that uses veneers, crowns, or other devices to change the shape of teeth is a high-end treatment that plumps the jaw and cheeks.

potential side effects include allergic reaction or lumps under the skin.

Topical lip plumpers (typically glosses) also offer temporary fullness to thinning lips, usually by irritating sensitive lip skin with stimulants such as mint, pepper, and menthol, and relying on moisturizers to hydrate lips and lend volume. Blue-based red and berry shades of lip color help yellowed teeth appear whiter, but keep it bright, since dark color calls attention to thinning lips. To keep color from migrating, trace lips with liner in the same shade as your lips.

Restore Your Pearly Whites to Their Younger Luster

Studies show that snacking on dairy foods, especially cheese, can preserve and even rebuild enamel. But limit sugary and acidic foods and drinks such as soda, fruit juices, coffee, and wine. When you do consume them, brush your teeth or rinse your mouth with water to wash away damaging acids and prevent enamel-eroding plaque and stains from forming.

Add a fluoride rinse after brushing to help strengthen enamel, use a soft-bristled toothbrush and fluoride toothpaste twice a day, and floss at least once daily. Overly vigorous brushing can cause gums to recede faster, so go easy, especially near your gum line. Like a little high-tech help? Some electric toothbrushes have a two-minute timer and a pressure-sensitive switch that shuts off if you're brushing too hard.

To combat the yellowing and stains that come with age, turn to tooth-whitening products. Whitening toothpastes use mild abrasives or chemicals to remove surface stains. To get at deeper stains, you'll need a bleaching treatment that uses carbamide peroxide or hydrogen peroxide. Inexpensive at-home versions with trays or strips require repeated applications and last about six months. Your dentist can make custom-fit trays for home use or perform an in-office treatment that takes an hour and lasts a year. The American Dental Association notes that teeth that have darkened to a brown or grayish color won't respond as well to bleaching treatments; if that's the case for you, talk to your dentist about porcelain veneers or dental bonding, which not only address discoloration but fix chips and cracks as well.

Age-Proof Your Hair

Strands of hair naturally get thinner and weaker with age. Research shows that after age forty, certain hair cells, called melanocytes, exhaust their ability to produce pigment, resulting in graying hair. DNA damage from smoking, sun exposure, and other factors can speed up that process, according to a 2009 study in the journal *Cell*. Hair loss due to heredity affects about thirty million American women and fifty million American men beginning as early as age thirty, although other factors, such as nutrition, medication side effects, and stress, can also cause hair to thin and fall out more rapidly. But your hair doesn't have to reveal your age. Here are some tricks to keep your tresses in top shape and instantly look younger.

Go Gray Gracefully—or Not

You might not think about protecting your hair from ultraviolet rays, especially outside of summer, but hair loses its natural UV defenses as it ages, and the resulting sun damage can speed up graying and make hair brittle and dull. Adding UV protection to your hair-care routine year-round can prevent that wear and tear, and if you've dyed your hair, can keep hair color from fading.

Whether you choose to color your salt and pepper strands or just keep them shiny and lustrous (read: younger-looking) is up to you. Gray hair is coarser and doesn't reflect light as well, and like the rest of your skin, your scalp produces less oil as you get older. Combined, these factors can lead to dry, dull hair that breaks easily. Restoring moisture and shine are key to turning back the clock. Try using moisturizing hair masks and deep conditioners when you color to protect hair and add shine and softness. If you're keeping your gray, look for shampoos and conditioners that cater to silver strands to prevent yellowing.

If you decide to dye, both semi-permanent and permanent dyes can add depth and make hair look fuller. But choose your colors carefully. Harsh, one-color dye jobs can age you, so opt for a dye that's within a few shades of your natural color, and add highlights to soften the look. And if you've been wearing your hair in the same style for the last decade, talk to your stylist about trying out a more modern look that adds volume. Once you hit forty, women should avoid too-long tresses (more than six inches past your shoulders) because heavy hair pulls on sagging skin, emphasizing wrinkles.

Halt Age-Related Hair Loss

If your hair loss is sudden or in a single spot, or if you suspect there's another

The Takeaway: Hair Helpers

Be gentle when styling; limit chemical processing; and avoid styles and styling tools that pull on hair (tight rollers, ponytails, weaves, braids, and uncoated rubber bands), which can permanently damage roots so they can no longer produce hair.

Shampoo every other day; switch to shampoos and conditioners with dimethicone (a shine enhancer) and cetyl alcohol (a hydrator).

Supplement your diet with vitamin B7 to halt hair loss.

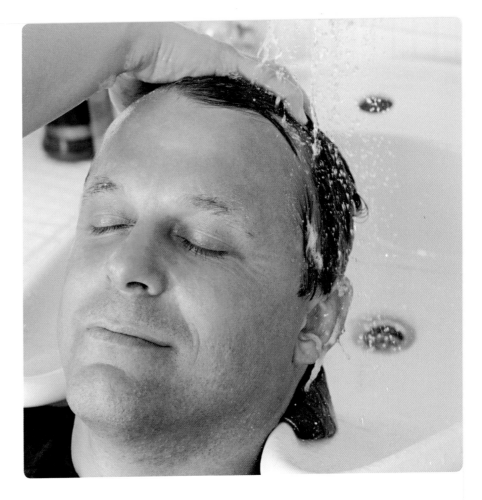

factor involved, like stress or medication side effects, see your dermatologist to determine the cause. For most people, hair loss is hereditary. To help slow it down, focus on nourishing and protecting your roots. First, exercise to boost circulation to your scalp, which stimulates follicles to grow healthy new hair. Next, feed your hair. Hair is made of protein, so load up on protein-rich foods, such as eggs or cottage cheese, to give hair the building blocks it needs. Biotin, or vitamin B7, forms the basis of hair cells, and a deficiency can cause brittleness or even hair loss. Good

sources of B7 include avocados, eggs, milk, nuts, and whole grains.

Although there is no research that shows high doses can reverse hair loss in healthy people, some dermatologists suggest supplementing with up to 5 milligrams biotin daily to give hair a boost (the U.S. Recommended Dietary Allowance [RDA] for biotin is 300 micrograms). It's nontoxic and inexpensive if you'd like to try it, but check with your doctor before popping a pill, since biotin may increase the effects of lipid-lowering medications. If you

need to bring in the big guns, topical minoxidil (Rogaine) and oral finasteride (Propecia) may help regrow hair or slow hair loss, but they carry side effects such as burning or stinging with minoxidil and even birth defects with finasteride, and both have to be used indefinitely to keep working.

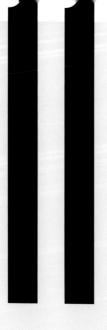

See a Dermatologist to Reduce Signs of Aging

Your dermatologist is a perfect partner as you try to fight the signs of aging skin. Besides having an annual examination to look for skin cancer, you can ask your dermatologist about all kinds of anti-aging products, treatments, and procedures, from antioxidant serums to Botox to a full-on face-lift. If you'd like more dramatic results than topical treatments can give you, but you're not ready to go under the knife, here are two popular in-office procedures that can take years off your appearance with very little downtime.

Lasers Lift Away Signs of Aging

Lasers first came on the scene as a way to resurface the skin in the 1980s, but the technology has continued to improve, leading to lasers that can repair sun damage like fine lines and discoloration, boost collagen production, and improve skin tone and firmness with a rapid recovery time. And unlike the original ablative carbon dioxide (CO_2) lasers, which damaged the top layer of skin (requiring about two weeks to heal) and carried the risk of scarring, the latest lasers have significantly less risk of side effects. The new wave includes nonablative and fractional lasers, and they work by using heat to damage the dermis, skin's lower layer, to stimulate healing and collagen production while leaving the surrounding skin and the epidermis intact. Both require a series of treatments for best results. A 2008 study in the *Journal of the American Academy of Dermatology* notes that nonablative lasers work best for treating early signs of aging, while fractional lasers are more effective for moderate wrinkles and sun damage.

One of the most popular new lasers is Fraxel, a fractional laser that requires three to six treatments at four- to six-week intervals for best results. Because it can be a little uncomfortable—some patients report it feels like a rubber band snapping against the skin—your dermatologist will likely apply a topical anesthetic to reduce pain before using the handheld device to go over the area to be treated. After the treatment, you might have a little swelling and a day or two of post-treatment redness. While Fraxel and other fractionated lasers won't erase deep wrinkles like CO_2 lasers can, they're a fantastic fix for fine lines, repairing sun damage, and improving skin tone and color. At the writing of this book, ablative laser treatments cost an average of $2,100, while nonablative lasers (including fractional) typically ran about $1,400, according to the American Society of Plastic Surgeons.

Wrinkle Fillers to the Rescue

Botox may get the most attention, but that muscle relaxer works best on forehead frown lines and isn't approved, or particularly effective, for wrinkles elsewhere on the face. For those—including deep creases—and for restoring lost volume to sunken cheeks or thinning lips, cosmetic fillers are your go-to treatments. Your dermatologist will inject a filler directly into the spot that needs plumping, bulking up the tissue underneath to provide smooth, firm support for skin. The most common fillers are collagen (Cosmoderm, Zyderm) and hyaluronic acid (Restylane, Juvéderm). Calcium hydroxylapatite (Radiesse) is another option that may also stimulate your skin's own collagen production. According to the American Society of Plastic Surgeons, results can last anywhere from two months to a year depending on the type of filler, with certain hyaluronic acid and calcium hydroxylapatite formulas being more likely to hit that yearlong mark. If you're looking for a longer-term fix, talk to your dermatologist about "very long duration" fillers such as fat cells or poly-L-lactic acid (Sculptra), which can last from one to three years.

You may want to pass on permanent fillers such as polymethyl methacrylate, or PMMA (ArteFill), since your face is always changing, and what looks good now may not be so flattering down the road. A 2008 study in the *Dermatology Online Journal* also noted that permanent fillers are "less forgiving and less versatile" than temporary fillers, and that people have more complications with permanent fillers, some of which can't be reversed even with surgery. If you opt for fillers of any kind, be sure to find a board-certified dermatologist or plastic surgeon who has experience using injectables, since skill and a good eye are required to use them well.

The Takeaway: Nonsurgical Procedures

New laser treatments reduce risks of scarring and recovery time while repairing moderate wrinkles and sun damage.

Botox works well on the forehead; other fillers plump the cheeks and lips.

Temporary fillers are a safer bet than permanent ones.

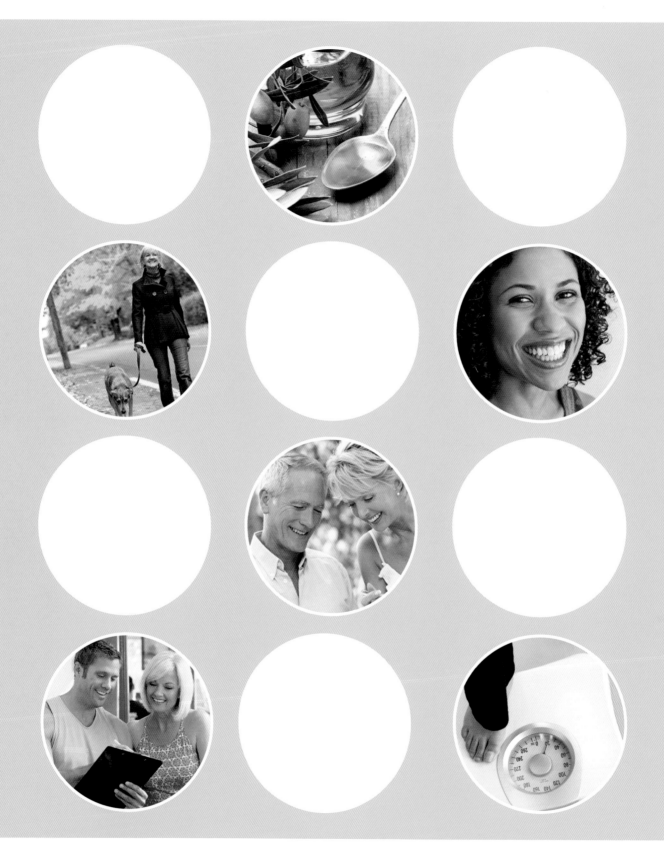

PART II

Turn Back the Clock on Your Figure

12

Rely on Math, Not a Magic Pill, to Keep a Youthful Figure

It's not as sexy as the latest diet craze sweeping through Hollywood, but in the search for a slimmer figure, slow and steady weight loss (one or two pounds a week) really does win the race. Whether you want to lose five pounds to fit into your clothes better or need to lose fifty to protect your health as you get older, losing weight boils down to a simple equation: The number of calories you take in must be less than calories out. In fact, diet plans that claim you don't need to count calories usually reduce your calorie intake anyway because you eat smaller portions or cut out certain foods (or in some cases, entire food groups). Some of those plans have helpful principles—reducing your refined-carb intake is almost always a healthy move, for instance (▶55)—but behind it all lies basic math. Even if you choose not to count calories, it's worth understanding a few key points about them.

Know Your Calorie Needs As You Age

Everyone has a baseline number of calories they need to maintain their current weight, but the number differs according to your gender, weight, activity level—and your age. It isn't just your imagination; your calorie needs do decline as you get older. Your metabolism slows about 5 percent each decade, so at age forty, women burn about 100 calories fewer per day and men burn about 50 calories fewer than they did at age thirty. That may not seem like much, but over a year it can translate to an extra five or ten pounds. The dip in your metabolism is mostly due to a decrease in muscle mass and a corresponding increase in body fat (▶21), but your organs also use fewer calories as you age.

The best way to determine your calorie quota is by measuring your resting metabolic rate (RMR), the number of calories your body requires for the daily tasks of living, such as breathing, blood circulation, and forming and repairing cells. Your gym may have a handheld device called a calorimeter that can measure your RMR pretty precisely. If you don't have access to a calorimeter, a 2005 review of studies in the *Journal of the American Dietetic Association* discovered that a tool called the Mifflin-St Jeor equation is the next most reliable way to estimate a person's RMR. You'll need to translate your weight from pounds to kilograms and height to centimeters; the formulas are as follows: 1 pound = 0.45 kg; 1 inch = 2.54 cm

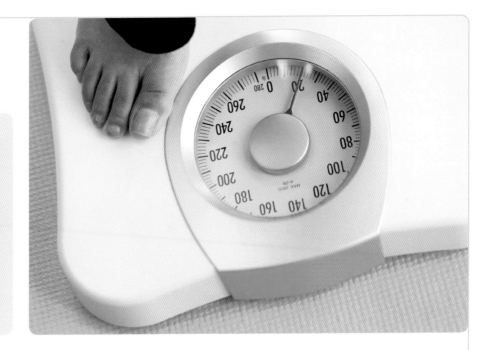

The Takeaway: The Weight Loss Equation

Losing one to two pounds per week will result in lasting weight loss.

Count calories and trim portions, but don't eat less than 1,200 calories a day or you'll actually slow your metabolism even more.

For men: (10 x weight in kg) + (6.25 x height in cm) – (5 x age in years) + 5

For women: (10 x weight in kg) + (6.25 x height in cm) – (5 x age in years) – 161

Once you have that number, you can add in your physical activity: Multiply your RMR by 1.3 if you're sedentary, 1.4 if you're moderately active, and 1.5 if you're very active. Although this number is just an estimate, it should give you a feel for how many calories you need to maintain your weight at your current activity level and fight the dreaded middle-age spread. To lose one pound a week, you'll have to create a deficit of 3,500 calories, or an average of 500 calories per day, from your RMR. It's easiest to reach that goal by both eating a little less and moving a bit more, but remember that it takes less time and effort to avoid eating 300 calories (a homemade cupcake) than it does to burn off the same amount through exercise (walking three miles at a 4-mph pace).

Don't Sabotage Your Anti-Aging Efforts with Crash Diets

Now that you know how many calories you need to burn to lose weight, it might be tempting to drastically limit your food intake to peel off pounds faster. But that strategy can backfire, say experts. Eating less than 900 calories a day sends your body into starvation mode and slows your metabolism by up to 20 percent. At that low intake, you'll also start burning precious muscle for energy, which makes your metabolism even more sluggish. Not to mention that it's nearly impossible to get the nutrition you need in that few calories. Don't go below 1,200 to 1,500 calories a day to keep your metabolism humming, ensure good nutrition, and burn fat instead of muscle.

13

Follow a Mediterranean Diet to Lose Weight and Live Longer

What makes the Mediterranean diet the healthiest anti-aging eating plan there is? A growing body of research confirms it's the diet's ability to help you drop pounds and add healthy years to your life. In 2009, Spanish researchers reviewed scientific studies on the diet and found some remarkable trends. Not only do people who eat a Mediterranean-style diet have longer life spans, they reduce their risk of cardiovascular disease, cancer, metabolic syndrome (a cluster of symptoms including belly fat, high cholesterol, high blood pressure, and high blood sugar), and even Alzheimer's and Parkinson's diseases. They also noted that the more closely the subjects followed a traditional Mediterranean diet (MD), the less likely they were to be obese. Additionally, a 2008 study in the *New England Journal of Medicine* found that people who followed the MD lost

more weight and had better blood sugar control than those who were on a traditional low-fat diet. What's more, sticking to the MD may be easier because it includes reasonable portions of healthy fats, which help you feel satisfied while eating less.

The Secret to a Longer Life Includes More than Olive Oil

Olive oil may be the most well-known component of the MD, but getting the most out of this eating style involves more than switching from butter to extra-virgin olive oil on your bread. The MD also incorporates fresh fruits and vegetables (on average, nine servings a day!), healthy fats such as olive oil and canola oil, whole grains, beans, fish or shellfish (at least twice a week), nuts and seeds, herbs and spices rather than salt, moderate amounts of red wine, and very little red meat. Bread, pasta, and

rice are all allowed, but refined sugars and processed foods are notably absent. Portion control also figures into the dietary equation, but since you're eating fresh, high-quality food, smaller portions can still satisfy.

The MD's emphasis on healthy fats may be its most distinguishing characteristic. While it includes little to no saturated fat or trans fats, the diet is rich in monounsaturated fats from olive oil, nuts, and avocados, and polyunsaturated fats such as omega-3s in fish. Besides increasing satiety (feelings of fullness), these fats confer considerable health benefits. Olive oil contains antioxidant compounds called phenols that help fend off free-radical damage to your DNA and calm inflammation that can accelerate aging. Omega-3s also offer a wealth of health benefits that can help you look and feel younger

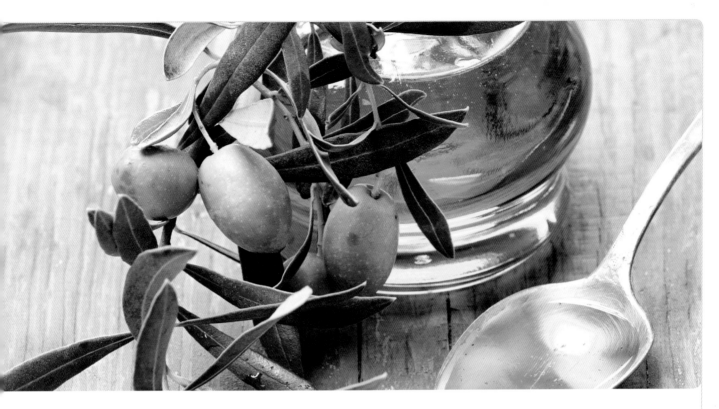

while protecting against age-related conditions like cognitive decline and heart disease (▶**25**, **58**).

The focus on fresh fruits and vegetables and nonmeat sources of protein also factors into the health and weight loss benefits of the diet. Mediterranean residents typically eat tomatoes, broccoli, peppers, capers, spinach, eggplant, mushrooms, white beans, lentils, and chickpeas, but all plant foods are on the table, so to speak. These foods are superb sources of antioxidants and other compounds that protect cells against the onslaught of aging. And because they're naturally low in calories and high in fiber, they can help you drop pounds without feeling deprived.

Reducing sweets and simple carbs is another key to the MD. Naturally sweet fruit is the dessert of choice in the Mediterranean region. Whole grains such as brown rice, polenta, barley, and whole-wheat couscous offer fiber and nutrients, and they won't spike your blood sugar like refined grains. A 2004 study in the *American Journal of Clinical Nutrition* also reported that men who increased their whole-grain intake were more likely to stave off middle-age weight gain. Overcoming decades of ingrained eating habits can be tough, so if eating this way feels totally foreign to you, start small—but do start.

The Takeaway: The Mediterranean Diet

Try making one meal a week according to MD principles. Buy a cookbook (or check out a few from the library), take a cooking class, or look at online recipe sites.

Update your favorite dishes to incorporate MD-friendly foods, such as adding beans, tomatoes, corn, and zucchini to your chili, while reducing the amount of meat called for.

Try simple swaps such as serving brown rice with your stir-fry and trading instant oatmeal for steel-cut oats in the morning.

14

Practice Portion Control to Offset an Aging Metabolism

You probably understand the concept of a serving of food: a commonly agreed-upon measure, like cups or tablespoons, that appears on the nutrition facts panel of packaged foods. A portion, however, is what you actually put on your plate. As your metabolism slows with age, understanding portions becomes even more critical to keeping your weight in check. It's a significant part of the Mediterranean diet (▶13) and can allow you to lose weight while you continue eating many of your favorite foods, ensuring you won't feel deprived. Research shows that people given large portions generally underestimate the number of calories foods contain—and our ability to count calories gets worse the larger the portions become. If you spend the time and effort to learn what a proper portion is, this strategy could just become one of your best tools to counteract a slowing metabolism.

Outsmart Your Midlife Metabolism by Retraining Your Brain

You might think that after several decades of eating, you have a good sense of what counts as a serving. Chances are, however, it's much smaller than you think. As restaurants have started supersizing dishes and more foods are available in bulk packs, our ability to estimate serving sizes has all but evaporated. The first step in correcting portion distortion is identifying what a serving of a food actually is. The USDA website mypyramid.gov lists serving sizes of common foods from all the major food groups. Next, when you start paying attention to portions, it helps to have measuring cups and spoons and a food scale at the ready. You won't need to rely on them forever—in fact, it may take as little as a week for your eyes

to recognize appropriate serving sizes, according to a 2009 study in the journal *Appetite*—but you should start by measuring every morsel you put in your mouth. Another trick is to try 100-calorie packs or to pre-portion foods that come in bigger packages so you're not tempted to mindlessly munch your way through several servings.

Commercially available dishes that visually indicate healthy portion sizes can also help. In fact, a study in the *Archives of Internal Medicine* found that using a specially designed plate and bowl that showed correct portions allowed midlife and older adults to lose significantly more weight over six months than those who didn't use the dishes. If you don't feel like carrying your measuring cups or your plate with you, using visual cues that match up to everyday objects can help you

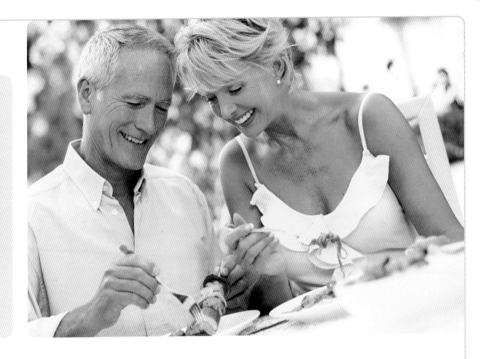

The Takeaway: Portion Control

You need less food as you age. Stick to the correct portions by using measuring cups or imagining comparable items: a deck of cards for meat or fish; a pair of dice for an ounce of cheese.

Trick your eyes by using smaller plates, and eat more slowly.

Pile your plate with low-calorie, high-volume foods like salads and broth-based soups.

judge accurately as well. For example, a medium orange and a small apple are both approximately the size of a baseball, a 1 ounce serving of cheese is the size of two dice, and a 3 ounce serving of meat compares to a deck of cards or the palm of your hand.

It will probably take some time to adjust to seeing less food on your plate, especially if you're still eating the same amount of food as you did in your twenties. One way to combat that, according to Cornell University food psychologist Brian Wansink, Ph.D., is to use smaller plates, effectively tricking your eyes into thinking you're eating more than you actually are. Wansink's research shows that even being aware of correct portion size isn't enough to counteract this powerful visual cue. In one study, people using a larger bowl to serve themselves cereal ended up

pouring and eating 16 percent more than people given smaller bowls. What's more, those given the smaller bowls actually estimated that they had gotten almost 8 percent more cereal than the others, increasing their sense of satisfaction despite eating less!

As You Age, Increase Satisfaction While Decreasing Intake

Eating less to counteract a slowing metabolism doesn't have to mean feeling hungry all the time. Eating more slowly can help you feel fuller with less food. Using chopsticks at mealtime is an effective way to slow you down, but you can also simply put your fork down between bites. Another way to increase your satisfaction is to pile your plate with lower-calorie foods that have more volume due to a higher air or water content. Fresh fruits and vegetables top this list (broth-based soups, popcorn,

and whipped potatoes also qualify), and many experts recommend loading half your plate with produce and dividing the rest between lean protein and complex carbohydrates.

15

Feast on Metabolism-Boosting Foods to Fight Middle-Age Spread

Besides making smart food choices (▶13) and practicing portion control (▶14), you can fight your body's natural decline in metabolism by eating foods that temporarily tip the scales in your favor by allowing you to burn extra calories. As your body digests, absorbs, and metabolizes food, it generates body heat—a process called thermogenesis that accounts for 10 to 15 percent of your daily calorie expenditure. A few foods are scientifically proven to increase thermogenesis by small amounts, thereby boosting calorie burn. Making them mainstays in your diet can help you shed unwanted pounds almost effortlessly.

Make It Hot to Boost an Aging Metabolism

A 2005 study in the *International Journal of Obesity* found that people ate up to 16 percent fewer calories over the course of two days when they consumed 0.9 grams of ground red pepper (a palatable amount) mixed into tomato juice before each meal. And the researchers noted that satiety increased even though the volunteers curbed their calorie intake. Spicy peppers from the capsicum family contain a compound called capsaicin, which gives those peppers their hotness. Around age fifty, you may start to lose taste buds, making flavors duller. Incorporating foods that provide the oral sensation of spiciness can intensify flavors and make eating more pleasurable, allowing you to turn up the heat at mealtime and get capsaicin's calorie-torching benefits. Studies show that capsaicin can help you shed pounds by spiking your metabolism and helping you eat less overall, partly by increasing feelings of fullness and partly because people tend to eat fiery foods more slowly, giving your brain more time to register that you're full. As another benefit of increased thermogenesis, capsaicin increases fat burning, which is especially beneficial as your body composition naturally shifts with age.

Research shows that nonpungent compounds called capsinoids from the same peppers are structurally similar to capsaicin, and animal studies suggest that they might also boost metabolism, although more research in humans is needed to verify this effect. Until we know more, pile on the hot peppers!

Count on Caffeine to Burn Calories As You Age

Not only does caffeine provide a pick-me-up for flagging energy levels as you get older, but studies show that as little as 50 milligrams can increase thermogenesis by up to 6 percent. Some research shows that epigallocatechin gallate (EGCG) compounds in green tea may make it an even better beverage for weight loss than coffee or other buzz-inducing drinks. In addition to EGCG's powerful antioxidant effects (which make it an anti-aging superstar), a 2010 review of studies in the *American Journal of Clinical Nutrition* showed that, compared with caffeine alone, green tea catechins plus caffeine decreased volunteers' BMIs by 0.55 and boosted weight loss by 3 pounds (1.38 kg). Not only that, but the combination shrank waistlines by about 0.75 inches (1.93 cm), making it a stellar choice to counteract your body's tendency to deposit fat around your middle as you get older (▶18). A 2009 study in the *International Journal of Obesity* found that caffeinated green tea not only helps you drop pounds, but it helps you keep them off as well.

If you're not a tea drinker, you can still get green tea's calorie-burning benefits in supplement form: Swiss researchers showed that taking green tea extract (50 milligrams caffeine and 90 milligrams EGCG) at breakfast, lunch, and dinner boosted calorie expenditure by 4 percent over twenty-four hours. That's almost enough to counteract the 5-percent-per-decade decrease in metabolism you experience with age (▶12).

Pick Protein to Preserve Metabolism-Boosting Muscle

Eating foods that both build muscle and burn calories can help you reverse age-related muscle loss (▶21) and keep a youthful figure. A 2008 study in the *American Journal of Clinical Nutrition* found that older men and women who consumed 20 percent of total calories from protein lost about 40 percent less muscle than those who ate the least protein (10 percent of their total calories). Protein helps muscles rebuild after exercise, adding muscle mass and increasing strength. It also takes more energy (read: calories) for your body to digest protein than carbs or fat, temporarily boosting your metabolism after you eat. Fish, lean meats, poultry, low-fat dairy, soy foods, legumes, nuts, and seeds are great sources; incorporate protein into each meal or snack for the most muscle-building benefits.

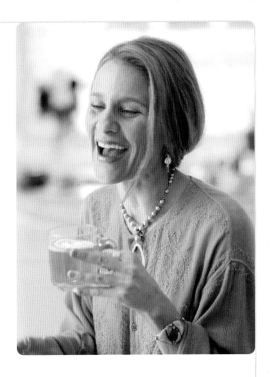

The Takeaway: Metabolism Boosters

Add ground red pepper and chile peppers to your diet to supercharge your metabolism.

Drink caffeinated drinks such as coffee and green tea to rev up your engine and whittle your waistline.

Eat lean proteins such as fish, poultry, soy, and nuts to build metabolism-maximizing muscle mass.

16

Eat Frequently to Stop Age-Related Weight Gain

Since you need fewer calories as you age (▶12), it might be tempting to skip meals or cut snacks to keep your weight in check. But if you miss breakfast, go too long without eating, or snack on sweets, you may not only set yourself up for diet disaster but speed up the aging process as well. You can snack your way to weight loss while getting the energy you need to do the things you love, keep cravings under control, and stay within your daily calorie budget. Here's how.

An Anti-Aging Diet Begins with Breakfast

Numerous studies show the benefits of eating breakfast—including helping you lose weight. People who skip breakfast actually tend to eat more calories overall (usually from sugary and fatty foods) throughout the day. And eliminating your morning meal likely means you're missing out on nutrients important to healthy aging. Of all the eating patterns examined by a 2006 study in the *Journal of the American Dietetic Association*, breakfast skippers had the lowest intakes of folic acid, vitamin C, calcium, magnesium, iron, potassium, and fiber—all critical for keeping your body, especially your bones and your cardiovascular system, young and healthy.

Besides helping to fill in nutritional gaps, a nourishing breakfast can jump-start your metabolism and cause you to burn calories at a higher rate all morning, helping to offset your body's natural metabolic decline as you get older. It can also set the stage for healthy eating all day by encouraging you to continue making wise food choices.

Many experts recommend seeing food as fuel, a mind-set backed up by a 2009 study in the *Journal of Nutrition* that found that women who ate a breakfast of muesli, yogurt, and fruit three hours before an hour-long walking workout burned 50 percent more fat than those who dined on cornflakes, white toast, and jam. The muesli meal also helped them feel fuller for the rest of the day, even though both breakfasts contained the same number of calories. Researchers noted that the difference was due to the protein, fiber, fat, and complex carbohydrates in the first breakfast, which fueled them with steady energy but didn't cause a spike in blood sugar.

Enlist These Snacking Strategies to Stay Young and Fit

To keep your total daily calorie intake in check, take a mini-meal approach. Research shows that eating five or six small meals a day (or three moderate meals and two snacks) keeps your

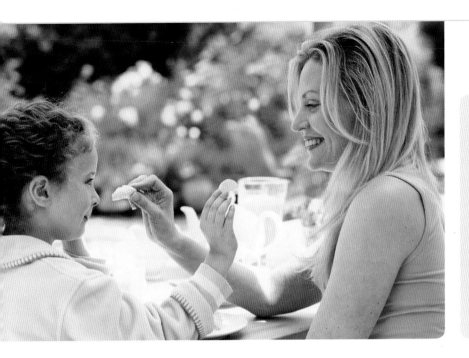

The Takeaway: Super Snacks

Eat small meals of 300 to 400 calories plus one or two 100- to 200-calorie snacks every three to four hours to keep your metabolism humming.

Combine protein with produce to make a power mini-meal: dried fruit and nuts, apple slices and peanut butter, or lettuce roll-ups with turkey and low-fat cheese.

blood sugar and energy levels steady and your metabolism humming. To lose weight, aim to eat every three to four hours, with meals measuring 300 to 400 calories and snacks weighing in at 100 to 200 calories, depending on your daily calorie needs.

But to make the mini-meal approach work, you may need to revise your definition of a snack. Dipping into your candy dish for an afternoon treat will backfire as your blood sugar comes crashing down, leaving you wiped out and craving more sugar. Refined carbohydrates, such as white flour, and sweets can also increase your insulin levels, raising your risk for diabetes, increasing belly fat (▶18), and aging your body. Choose complex carbohydrates, such as whole grains, instead, and make sure all your meals and snacks contain protein and a little healthy fat to keep

your blood sugar steady and help you stay full longer. For example, top half a 100-percent whole-wheat English muffin with a slice of Cheddar and tomato, or dip vegetables in white bean spread drizzled with a little olive oil. Protein is also critical for holding on to metabolism-boosting lean muscle mass as you get older (▶15, 21); include some every time you eat to ensure you get enough.

Another principle of smart snacking is to sneak in more fruits and vegetables. It can be tough to get the recommended five to nine servings of produce per day through meals alone, but building your snacks around fruits and veggies is a delicious, low-calorie way to help you reach your goal and reap the benefits of their age-fighting antioxidants and protective compounds. Bonus: It's hard to binge on baby carrots. World-class snacks that meet these criteria include

apple slices with low-fat string cheese, an orange and one ounce of almonds, celery sticks spread with one tablespoon of peanut butter, plain nonfat yogurt with berries and granola, and red pepper slices with a few tablespoons of hummus.

17

Sip Selectively to Stay Slim and Trim for a Lifetime

Research shows that your brain doesn't register liquid calories as well as those from solid food, so you can drink a full meal's worth of calories and still not feel full. A recent review of studies suggested that substituting water and other calorie-free quenchers (diet soft drinks, coffee, and tea) for soda, juice, and alcohol may help people reach and stay at a healthy weight. And a surprising 2009 study in the *American Journal of Clinical Nutrition* found that cutting calories from sugar-sweetened beverages helped participants lose more weight than trimming calories from solid food. Since sugar promotes fat storage around your middle as you get older (▶18), making better beverage choices may not only result in a lower number on the scale, but it may help reshape your figure and prevent or reverse the stereotypical middle-age spread.

You'll need to sip selectively to avoid empty calories, but you don't have to forgo all your favorite drinks. For example, make your latte a lot leaner by switching to nonfat milk, shunning whipped cream, and asking for a smaller amount of flavored syrups. Better yet, ditch the syrup entirely and sprinkle cocoa or cinnamon on top for guilt-free flavor. Alcohol is a sneaky source of extra calories, and cocktail mixers can really tip the scale. If you choose to imbibe, your best bet is a 5 ounce glass of wine, which contains about 110 calories.

Make Water Your Anti-Aging Beverage of Choice

If you're looking for one simple diet tweak to offset your naturally slowing metabolism as you get older, drinking more water could be your golden ticket. A 2005 study in the journal *Obesity*

Research found that people who were regular water drinkers—meaning they drank about 52 ounces (1.53 L) per day, on top of milk, juice, and the occasional soft drink—consumed an average of 193 fewer calories a day than people who didn't drink any water. Think water is too boring? Add a twist of lemon or lime, or add fresh berries to a pitcher of water and keep it in the fridge to infuse it with calorie-free flavor. If you want to add fizz for extra interest, make your own sparkling water with a seltzer bottle (aka a soda siphon) and carbon dioxide cartridges. Or use your water to make tea, which has other health and weight loss benefits (▶15).

Starting your meal with a glass of water can also help you eat less, according to a 2008 study in the *Journal of the American Dietetic Association*. In the study, a group of sixty-year-old adults who drank 500 ml (a little over 2 cups) of water thirty minutes before breakfast ate 13 percent fewer calories during the meal than those who didn't drink water. Interestingly, researchers in the same lab published a related study that showed this effect was true for older adults (sixty to eighty years old), but not for adults younger than thirty-five.

Make Friends with Fiber to Banish Midlife Flab

If you're a fan of fruit juice, switch to 100 percent juice varieties that contain pulp to get a little satiating fiber with no added sugar. Of course, whole fruit is still your best bet, but if you're thirsting for a drink, whip up a fruit smoothie using chunks of frozen fruit and a little juice or milk. For an extra dose of filling fiber, toss in a handful of oats or a tablespoon of wheat germ or ground flaxseed. That simple addition may also help combat your body's tendency to store fat around your middle as you get older—a 2007 study in the *American Journal of Clinical Nutrition* found that people who ate the most whole grains and cereal fiber had lower BMIs and smaller waistlines (by two-and-a-half inches!) than those who ate the least.

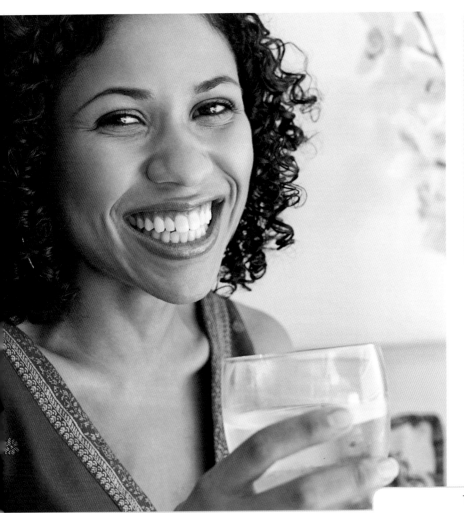

The Takeaway: Smart Sips

Make water your beverage of choice.

Gradually reduce the amount of sugar you stir into your tea or coffee.

Mix your lemonade into unsweetened tea to make a homemade Arnold Palmer that slashes calories in half without sacrificing taste.

Stir some fiber into a fruit smoothie to slim your waistline.

18

Escape the Stress-Fat Cycle for a More Youthful Waistline

As you get older, your body naturally starts to deposit more fat around your middle. Men physically have more fat cells in their abdomens, so their bodies prefer to store extra pounds there. For women, declining estrogen levels in midlife signal fat to start accumulating around the waist as well. Having some fat inside your abdomen is normal, and in fact, it is your body's main source of energy when you face fight-or-flight stress. But long-term—or chronic—stress continually floods your body with high levels of the stress hormone cortisol. That causes you to gain too much belly fat, which in turn raises your risk of cardiovascular disease, high blood pressure, high cholesterol, diabetes, and even cancer. The kicker? Weight gain that results from stress is stubborn and will resist your best efforts at eating healthfully and exercising. To lose your stress fat, especially after age forty, try

these tips to become more resilient and put a stop to stress eating.

Beat the Midlife Stress-and-Food Double Whammy

Stress can affect your eating habits in several ways. For some people, both positive and negative stress—whether it's an important work deadline, planning your child's wedding, a chronic health condition, or caring for aging parents—can trigger overeating. Food acts as both a comfort and a distraction. For others, responsibilities can get so overwhelming that they go for too long without eating, and then grab anything they can get their hands on. In both situations, cortisol is at work. In 2009, researchers at the University of Michigan found that higher levels of cortisol prompted people to take in more calories and food overall. A 2007 study in the journal *Nutrition* noted that chronic stress makes you more likely

to reach for sugary, fatty foods, possibly because they provide more energy (in the form of calories) to deal with anxiety-inducing events. Sweet, rich foods also activate a release of feel-good chemicals called endorphins that act almost like a drug in your system to calm the stress response and improve mood.

But breaking out the brownies can backfire—refined carbs cause a rapid spike and fall in blood sugar, wreaking havoc with insulin levels as they try to restore balance, triggering further cravings, and promoting fat storage in your abdomen. With this chain reaction in place, it's no surprise that stress can make you pile on pounds. Unfortunately, the diet and exercise regimen that worked in your youth won't be as effective to help you lose weight as you age: You now have to add in a stress management component.

Stress-Proof Your Days for Longer Life (and a Slimmer Figure)

Even with the cortisol connection and metabolic changes working against you, however, an after-forty expanding waistline is not inevitable. Even minor tweaks to tame tension can make a big difference. For example, if you eat for comfort, stop stressed-out snacking by creating a list of nonfood, feel-better treats you can turn to in the face of anxiety, such as buying fresh flowers or getting a massage. Boost your mood by putting down the doughnut and lacing up your sneakers to raise your endorphin levels. Exercise attacks stress fat on both fronts: Not only does it burn calories, but also it's a surefire stress reliever. Research shows that even a ten-minute walk can improve your outlook and help you regain perspective.

Taking the initiative to address your stressors is also helpful, since much of our stress comes from feeling like things are out of our control. This can be especially true in mid- and later life, as family relationships and work life veer off into uncharted territory. Try identifying the specific stressor in a situation and picking a response that directly counters it. Navigating a newly empty nest? Tackle loneliness by blocking out time to connect with friends, current or former coworkers, or a neighbor you've been meaning to introduce yourself to. Dealing with a sticky family situation? If you're feeling helpless, ask trusted friends for advice and a sense of solidarity. Planning for retirement got you on edge? If you're concerned about money, make an appointment with a financial advisor to take stock of what you have and set up a budget.

The Takeaway: Stress and Belly Fat

It's normal for your waistline to expand after age forty. In women, declining estrogen levels lead to greater fat stores at the waist; men have more fat cells there to begin with.

Stress adds to belly fat by leading you to overeat, especially with sugary and/or fatty foods such as cookies and chips.

Take control of stress by identifying long-term stressors and relieving tension with noncaloric treats.

19

Lose Weight by Addressing Age-Related Sleep Changes

Can you lose weight while you sleep? It's not just a dream—an increasing body of evidence shows that sleep plays a role in weight gain and obesity. In particular, researchers have recently turned their attention to two hormones that control appetite: ghrelin and leptin. Ghrelin, produced in your gastrointestinal tract, triggers hunger. Leptin is produced in fat cells and tells your brain when you're full. And sleep affects the production of both.

As you get older, your sleep habits may change. Studies show that circadian rhythms, which manage your sleep/wake cycle, shift with age. That's why even former night owls frequently find themselves going to bed and waking up earlier, spending less time in deep sleep, and sleeping less overall. And according to the National Sleep Foundation, up to 80 percent of older adults with four or more health problems report not sleeping well. These changes, combined with an increased risk of insomnia and sleep disorders as you get older, can throw off ghrelin and leptin levels, frustrating even the best-laid weight loss plans. (Studies also show that estrogen affects ghrelin production, so women in midlife may have an even harder time, thanks to fluctuating hormones.)

Too little sleep disrupts the hormonal balance in two ways. It lowers leptin levels, meaning you don't register the feeling of fullness that signals you to stop eating. But it also raises ghrelin levels, which can make you ravenous. University of Chicago researchers examined the ghrelin and leptin levels of twelve men after two days of restricted sleep and then two days of extended sleep. Not only did they find that the men's ghrelin levels were higher and leptin levels lower after sleep restriction, making them hungrier, but the men also had cravings for high-calorie, high-carb foods. A 2009 study in the *American Journal of Clinical Nutrition* tried a similar approach, restricting the sleep of middle-aged men and women to just 5.5 hours a night for two weeks. They found that the volunteers took in about 300 more calories from high-carb snacks per day than they did during a two-week period when they slept for 8.5 hours. Even more revealing, Stanford researchers looked at the sleep habits of more than one thousand people and found that the less sleep they got, the higher their BMI.

The Insulin Connection to Midlife Obesity

In 2010, researchers at the University of Chicago reviewed studies noting the connection between lack of sleep and obesity. In addition to the ghrelin-

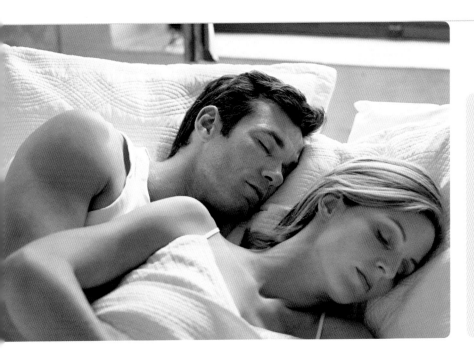

The Takeaway: Sleep Matters

Quality sleep regulates the hormones that trigger hunger and feelings of fullness.

Lack of sleep increases cravings for high-carb foods and triggers excess production of insulin, leading to belly fat and possibly diabetes.

Sleep problems increase as you get older, so practice good sleep habits to ensure you get enough rest.

leptin link, they found that not getting enough shut-eye can reduce insulin sensitivity. Insulin helps your cells use blood sugar (glucose) for fuel and also converts calories into fat. As your body becomes less sensitive, your pancreas has to pump out increasingly greater levels of insulin to make sure your cells get enough glucose and to keep your blood sugar normal. That extra insulin also means more calories get stored as fat, and as you get older, the double whammy of insulin and aging makes it more likely that the fat gets stored in your abdomen (▶18). Ultimately, this nasty cycle raises your risk for type 2 diabetes, which accelerates aging in almost all of your body's systems (▶55).

Snooze to Lose Pounds for Life

Sleep timing, duration, and quality all play a role in keeping your hormones balanced. Try to doze off and wake up at approximately the same time every day, including weekends. To reset your sleep schedule, gradually head to bed fifteen minutes earlier and/or set your alarm for fifteen minutes later, until you've carved out seven or eight hours for sleeping. Light signals your brain that it's time to sleep or wake up, so about an hour before bedtime, dim the lights. Keep your bedroom dark at night; purchase light-blocking shades if necessary. As you get older, nighttime bathroom breaks frequently increase; install a night-light to avoid using the bright overhead light, which can make falling asleep again harder. In the morning, open your shades to let in sunlight.

If you already get enough sleep and still feel tired (and hungry) all the time, ask your doctor if you might have obstructive sleep apnea. Your risk increases as you get older, so it's worth looking into even if you've never had problems sleeping in the past. Apnea can cause you to stop breathing for short periods, sometimes hundreds of times a night. This disrupts your sleep and can leave you feeling groggy during the day even if you spent eight or nine hours in bed.

20

Get Your Heart Pumping to Rev Up Midlife Metabolism

Whether you walk, hike, run, dance, skate, cycle, row, swim, or ski, aerobic activity will help you lose weight and offset the natural decline in metabolism as you get older. Not only do you burn calories during exercise, but your metabolism stays elevated after you finish working out. Exercise can also whittle your waistline, which helps you look younger and will keep you healthy long-term (▶18). In fact, a 2006 study in the journal *Obesity Reviews* noted that studies using imaging techniques to measure abdominal fat showed that exercise significantly reduced the amount of that particular health-threatening pudge even before subjects saw changes in overall body weight or waist measurements.

As you age, you lose lean muscle mass (▶21). And while shedding pounds through diet alone does reduce body

fat, it also triggers a further loss of muscle, which ultimately undermines your metabolism. Adding exercise to the equation, however, sets you up for success. Researchers at the University of Pittsburgh School of Medicine found that walking at a moderate intensity three to five times per week for thirty-five to forty-five minutes helped adults in their sixties and early seventies hold on to metabolism-boosting muscle.

The National Institute on Aging suggests aiming for at least thirty minutes of moderate-intensity aerobic activity on most or all days of the week, along with strength, balance, and flexibility exercises. If you're new to exercise, talk to your doctor about what kind of activity is best for you and how you can safely start moving and work up to that thirty-minute goal.

Work Out to Boost Your Metabolism As You Get Older

Any exercise is better than nothing, and as little as ten minutes can stoke your calorie-burning furnace. Still, don't just take a stroll around the block and hang up your sneakers. You'll see more metabolism improvements if you pick up the pace and go a little longer. (Always warm up and cool down with a few minutes of light activity to prevent injury and allow you to push yourself a little harder during your workout.) Exercising vigorously—at about 80 percent of your maximum heart rate (calculate your maximum heart rate by subtracting your age from 220)—burns the most calories in a session, but check with your doctor to determine a safe range. And duration matters too: If you exercise for more than fifteen minutes, you'll blaze through your body's glycogen stores and start using fat for fuel. Research also

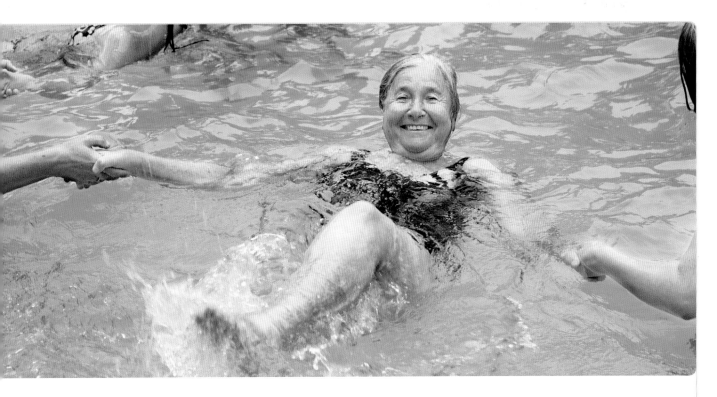

shows that working out longer and at a higher intensity keeps your metabolism fired up longer than a shorter, less strenuous sweat session, burning more calories even while you're at rest.

A 2009 study in the journal *Metabolic Syndrome and Related Disorders* found that in older adults who were not dieting to lose weight, high-intensity exercise (about 75 percent of their aerobic capacity) was more effective than moderate exercise in reducing belly fat. However, if you're also cutting calories to lose weight, moderate-intensity exercise may still do the trick by slimming you down all over, according to a study in the *American Journal of Clinical Nutrition*. In that study, both moderate and vigorous exercise helped subjects preserve muscle during weight loss—a key to keeping your metabolism fired up.

To keep your metabolism humming, variety is critical. Modify your exercise routine from time to time to challenge new muscles, or add in a few sprint-like bursts of activity to burn more calories and fat without feeling like you're working harder overall (▶94). You can alter the length of your workouts as well, which not only helps you fit in exercise when you have time, but also allows you to focus on different benefits: An intense twenty-minute workout will torch calories, for instance, while a long, steady workout boosts endurance and burns more fat. Variety also helps you beat boredom and reduces your risk of injury, ensuring that you can stay active.

The Takeaway: Metabolism Boosters

Amp up your workouts to keep your metabolism high even as you rest.

Aim for thirty minutes of moderate-to-vigorous aerobic exercise on most days of the week.

Vary your exercise routines to stoke your metabolism and keep boredom at bay.

21

Weight Train to Reverse Muscle Loss As You Get Older

After age forty-five, you lose about 1 percent muscle mass per year, or a half pound, and gain fat in its place. Not surprisingly, research also shows that with that loss of muscle comes loss of strength, which may prevent you from doing activities you enjoy. Muscle is metabolically active, meaning that it requires calories to function, and the amount of muscle you have significantly affects your resting metabolic rate (▶12). Since one pound of muscle uses between 35 and 50 calories a day just to maintain itself, losing five pounds of muscle over a decade may reduce resting metabolism by 175 to 250 calories a day. And without that muscle to maintain, the extra calories you consume get stored as fat.

The only way to reverse muscle decline is to build muscle through exercise and strength training. The good news is

that you can see results pretty quickly. Studies show that previously inactive older adults who start a strength training program can gain up to three pounds of muscle in just three months, boosting metabolism by about 7 percent and muscle strength by 50 percent. And if you're cutting calories to keep your weight in check, resistance training helps preserve muscle while you shed pounds, ensuring that the weight you lose comes from fat.

A Strength Training Program to Regain Youthful Muscle

To build muscle, you'll need to do strength exercises at least twice a week for thirty minutes or more, in addition to doing aerobic exercise for at least thirty minutes on most days of the week. Take at least one day off between strength sessions to let muscles rest and rebuild. A solid strength training program

includes exercises that address all your major muscle groups: chest, upper back, shoulders, biceps, triceps, quadriceps (quads), hamstrings and glutes, calves, and abdominal muscles. The Mayo Clinic website features a slide show of basic exercises that work most of these muscles, with pictures and written instructions: www.mayoclinic.com /health/weight-training/SM00041.

In general, start with light weights that allow you to perform an exercise with good form (where you can maintain the proper body position and control the weight) at least eight times in a row. If you can't, switch to a lighter weight. If that feels easy to you, trade up to a heavier weight. For each repetition (rep), focus on making your movements smooth and controlled, taking three seconds to lift, holding for one second, and then taking another three seconds to return to your starting position. Aim for ten to fifteen reps per exercise, to make up one set. Research shows that training with single or multiple sets produces similar strength gains, provided you use a heavy enough weight that you feel fatigued at the end of a set. If you decide to do a single set, therefore, you may need to use a slightly heavier weight to reach that point. When doing multiple sets, rest for at least two minutes in between to allow your muscles to refresh their energy resources.

You don't need a gym membership to put together a challenging strength routine. Many effective exercises, such as lunges, squats, push-ups, and crunches, rely on your body weight for resistance. If you invest in a good pair of shoes and some dumbbells and/or resistance bands, you can do most exercises (or similar modifications) at home without any other equipment. If you're looking to build a home gym, you might want to add an adjustable weight bench as well.

As with aerobic exercise, variety is key to successful strength training. Working your muscles from different angles targets more muscle fibers, helping to develop the muscles more completely and maximizing strength. Varying the exercises you do also keeps your muscles from getting used to the familiar movements and ensures that you'll continue seeing results from your efforts. Changing the amount of weight you use or the number of reps is an easy way to mix up your routine, or you can try new exercises and incorporate new weight machines or fitness tools. Fitness magazines and exercise videos can help you expand your repertoire of moves and suggest new ways to challenge your muscles.

The Takeaway: Strength Training

After age forty-five, you lose about a half pound of muscle per year. The calories that muscle used to burn instead get stored as fat.

Weight training is the only way to rebuild muscle. Older adults who start a strength training program can gain three pounds of muscle in three months.

Do strength exercises at least twice a week for thirty minutes, in addition to aerobic exercise.

22

Be Active in Your Free Time to Fight Metabolism Slowdown

Your body burns calories in three ways: performing the necessary functions of living (resting metabolic rate [▶12]), digesting food, and moving around, which is scientifically referred to as activity thermogenesis. Activity thermogenesis includes all the movement you do in a day, from your half-hour morning jog to brushing your teeth at night. While you know that sustained exercise can boost your metabolism (▶20, 21), small bursts of activity throughout the day also burn calories and help keep your metabolism fired up. These everyday movements are called nonexercise activity thermogenesis, or NEAT, and they actually make up the bulk of your daily calorie expenditure, according to James Levine, M.D., Ph.D., a scientist who has studied NEAT extensively.

Researchers are beginning to redefine what a sedentary lifestyle is. If you exercise in the morning but have a desk job and don't get up from your computer except maybe for lunch and the occasional bathroom break, that actually qualifies as a sedentary lifestyle. If you then drive home and spend a few hours in front of the TV… well, you can see why increasing NEAT can make a big difference.

A slew of studies show that calories used in NEAT activities can quickly offset the natural decline in your metabolism. Researchers at the Mayo Clinic found people do less NEAT activity as they get older, so intentionally adding it back in can help you stay active, trim, and young. This kind of activity also helps you hold on to your functional ability so you can continue doing things you enjoy—such as playing hide-and-seek with your grandkids, carrying your groceries from the car to inside, hoisting your suitcase into the overhead compartment, and climbing stairs—much longer than you would otherwise.

Stand Up for Weight Loss over Time

A landmark 2005 study in the journal *Science* measured the movements of twenty volunteers—ten lean and ten mildly obese—over the course of ten days and found that, on average, the obese volunteers were seated for a full two hours longer per day than their lean counterparts. The researchers, including Levine, noted that if they would adopt the NEAT behaviors the lean volunteers employed, the obese individuals could burn up to 350 calories more per day, even without formally "exercising"!

NEAT might be the most underused tool in your weight loss arsenal, but it's easy to reap the benefits. For example, a woman who needs to burn 100 calories more per day than she did ten years ago could knock them out simply by playing a Wii Sports game instead of watching TV for an hour. Basically, your goal is to break out of sedentary behaviors, interrupting them with periods of activity. Even standing occasionally to break up long spans of sitting can help—one reason why experts recommend delivering news to a coworker in person rather than via email. If you start to look, you can find plenty of opportunities to sneak activity into your chair-centric everyday life.

One way to increase NEAT is by adding movement to normally stationary activities, like pacing or doing dishes while you talk on the phone, or folding clothes while you watch the evening news. (Chores and yard work in general are an excellent opportunity to get moving, since they are usually physical in nature.) And a few minutes here and there of extra activity pay off without much effort at all. You've probably heard the suggestions to park farther away from the entrance and take the stairs instead of the elevator. You can also take the dog for a walk instead of letting him out in the backyard, dust and vacuum one room a day instead of using

a cleaning service, swap dinner and a movie for a trip to the museum, cook dinner instead of ordering in, do a few biceps curls while you're waiting for Web pages to load, and even put often-used items out of reach so you have to stand up to get them. You get the idea—anytime you find yourself sitting, think about how you can make that time more active. And there's a cyclical effect: Levine's research shows that increasing NEAT activities significantly increases energy, spurring you to incorporate even more metabolism-boosting movement into your day.

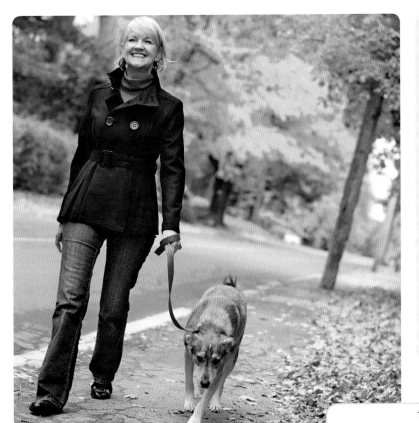

The Takeaway: Activity Bursts

Nonexercise activity thermogenesis (NEAT) makes up the bulk of your calorie expenditure. Find ways to increase your daily NEAT, such as walking or biking to nearby locations instead of driving, pacing or doing chores while you talk on the phone, and taking the dog for a walk around the block.

Move around more, even if you have a desk job: Get up for a few minutes every hour to get a drink of water or visit a coworker; use the stairs instead of the elevator; and deliver news in person rather than by email.

23

Focus on Flexibility and Core Work to Maintain Balance As You Age

In addition to aerobic exercise and strength training, flexibility and balance exercises should earn a spot on your to-do list for staying young and healthy. As you get older, your muscles become less elastic and tissues around your joints get thicker, which makes movement more difficult. If you don't take action to counteract this, you can lose 10 percent of your flexibility every ten years. Incorporating stretching into your exercise routine gives you more freedom of movement and makes daily activities like bending down, getting dressed, and reaching for something on a high shelf much easier. Staying flexible can also help you maintain balance; prevent falls; relieve chronic pain and tension; and improve circulation, mental focus, and energy. Just think about how good it feels to stretch after sitting in a chair for a long time!

Balance work is also a critical addition to your anti-aging fitness plan. Research confirms that your sense of balance declines with age, partly because of reduced muscle strength and control. The National Institute on Aging estimates that more than one-third of people age sixty-five or older fall each year. Falls and related injuries, such as breaking a hip, can limit your activities or keep you from living independently. Balance and strength exercises, particularly for your core abdominal muscles and lower body, are key to preventing falls because they give you more control over your body, keep your muscles strong, and improve your coordination.

Stretch Yourself to Age Gracefully

You'll get the most flexibility benefits by purposefully stretching your muscles at least three times a week; adding stretching sessions to your other workouts is often convenient, since your muscles are already warmed up. You should stretch all your major muscle groups: calves, quadriceps and hamstrings, hip flexors, chest, and upper back. You also can stretch your neck, shoulders, wrists, and ankles. Always warm up first, since stretching a cold muscle can raise your risk of pulling it. Don't force the stretch or bounce, but slowly and smoothly ease into the stretch, keeping your joints slightly bent, and hold it for at least thirty seconds. Be sure to breathe normally throughout. Repeat each stretch three to five times, and try to reach a little further each time. You might feel a little discomfort as you extend your reach, but you should stop if you feel pain. You can stretch periodically throughout the day if that makes it easier to fit it in, or you can set aside a block of time to stretch your whole body. Exercises like yoga,

Pilates, tai chi, and resistance stretching (a technique that over-forty Olympian Dara Torres uses in her training) combine multiple benefits of flexibility, balance, and strength.

Exercise for Better Balance Late in Life

You can do balance exercises just about anywhere, but when you start, make sure you have a wall or chair nearby in case you become unsteady. Start by supporting yourself with both hands, then remove one hand, try supporting yourself with just one finger, and finally let go. If you're steady on your feet, you can increase the challenge by doing the exercises with your eyes closed. The National Institute on Aging recommends basic balance exercises such as standing on one foot, walking heel to toe, and walking with slow, exaggerated steps in a straight line with your arms stretched out to your sides. You can also try standing up from a seated position without using your hands, one-legged squats, and many upper-body exercises (like biceps curls) while standing on one foot. All of these exercises engage small muscles in your abdominal core to keep you upright and steady. A few fitness tools, such as stability balls, Bosu balls, wobble boards, balance disks, and even a pillow can help you improve your balance. You can do specific balance exercises on them, but doing traditional moves like crunches, squats, and push-ups with them is also beneficial because they engage your core, challenge your muscles in new ways, and make you work harder to maintain balance.

The Takeaway: Flexibility and Balance

Unless you counteract the natural aging process, you'll lose 10 percent of your flexibility every ten years.

Stretch twice a week to prevent falls, relieve pain and tension, and improve circulation.

An easy way to boost balance is to do upper-body exercises while standing on one foot.

24

Tools and Tips for a Younger Metabolism

Eating reasonable portions of nourishing foods, combating stress, getting enough sleep, and exercising regularly are cornerstones of healthy weight loss, and they will all help counteract the natural slowdown in your metabolism as you get older. If you've adopted those behaviors and you're still not seeing the scale budge, or if you've reached a plateau, some small tweaks are in order. These smart strategies can help you master your metabolism and stay healthy, fit, and trim for the rest of your life.

Track Your Midlife Body Fat Percentage

You know the importance of maintaining a healthy weight as you get older (▶41, 53). But your scale doesn't give you the full picture. Muscle burns up to three times as many calories as fat, so a 130-pound woman with 25 percent body fat (a healthy range) will burn about 200 more calories per day than a 130-pound woman with 40 percent body fat (a typical amount for midlife). Even if you are at a healthy weight, if your body fat is too high, you could have a condition called normal-weight obesity, which carries many of the same health risks as obesity. Since your body composition naturally shifts as you get older (▶12), it's increasingly important to keep tabs on your body fat as well as the number on the scale.

Your mirror and the way your clothes fit are helpful gauges, but the most accurate way to measure your body fat percentage is to find an exercise physiologist or certified trainer who can perform a body fat analysis. Your local gym or a hospital-affiliated fitness center should have a person on staff or be able to direct you to someone trained to do the analysis. According to National Institutes of Health recommendations, the healthy body fat range for women between ages forty and fifty-nine is 23 to 35 percent, and 24 to 36 percent for those over sixty. The healthy ranges in men aged forty to fifty-nine are 11 to 22 percent, and 13 to 25 percent for those over sixty. Get rechecked every three months or so to track your progress. Handheld devices and scales with built-in body fat analyzers are generally not very accurate because they depend on so many factors, such as how hydrated you are when you take the measurement. They may help you spot general upward and downward trends, however, so they can be useful tools as long as you understand their limitations.

Track Your Diet and Exercise to Outsmart a Sluggish Metabolism

Your memory is notoriously unreliable when estimating your food intake. It's easy to forget the handful of M&Ms you swiped from a coworker's candy dish or overlook your "samples" while cooking dinner. But those little bites add up, and they're especially critical to note because you need fewer calories now than you used to. Keeping track of your food intake in a journal or computer program can help you judge not only how many calories you're taking in, but the overall quality of your diet as well.

In the same vein, logging your exercise might also reveal a few surprises. You may notice that you're only doing one workout a week that's longer than twenty minutes, for example, or that exercise is always the first thing to go when you're under pressure. Seeing those patterns in black and white can help you pinpoint problem areas and brainstorm realistic solutions.

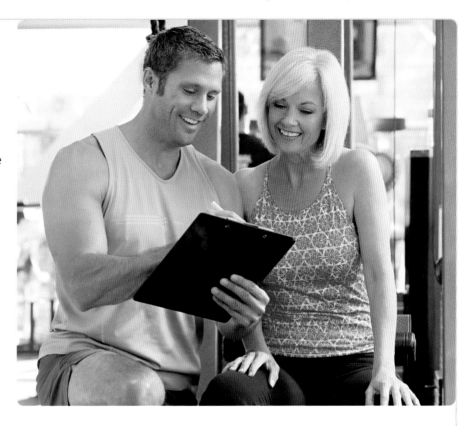

Set Reachable Anti-Aging Goals and Reward Yourself

Rewards are a powerful motivator, but they're most effective when you break down your overarching goals into specific, doable steps, especially if you're trying to overcome decades-old behaviors. For example, try eating one more fruit and vegetable a day or adding an extra ten minutes to one workout a week. Simply seeing a row of gold stars next to your food and exercise journal may be enough to motivate you to stay on track. External rewards can reinforce positive choices as well. Try setting aside $5 every time you work out. You can use the money to buy a small treat at the

end of the week (new music, flowers, a book), or a larger reward at the end of the month (new exercise clothes, a course in something you've wanted to learn). If you exercise five times a week for a year, you'll have $1,300—enough to take a vacation or invest in a piece of home gym equipment.

The Takeaway: Track Your Metabolism

Check your body fat every three months. Even if your weight on the scale is in the normal range, if your body fat is over 36 percent (for women) or 25 percent (for men), you risk having obesity-related health problems.

Put your numbers down on paper: exactly what you eat (and when and why), plus how often and how long you exercise. The trends may surprise you.

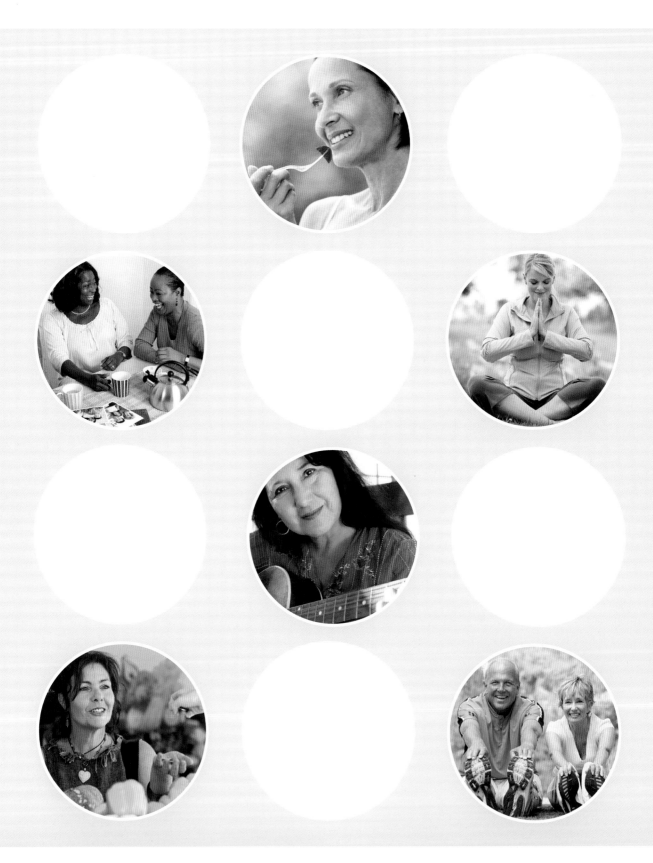

PART III

Turn Back the Clock on Your Brain

25

Eat an Anti-Inflammatory Diet to Keep Your Brain Young

The bad news is that your risk of dementia (including Alzheimer's disease) and other cognitive problems increases as you get older. The Cleveland Clinic notes that you have about a 5 percent chance of experiencing dementia when you're sixty-five, and the risk doubles every five years after that. The good news is that research shows you can do a lot to keep your brain healthy and young—including eating an anti-inflammatory diet. Inflammation is a factor in many chronic diseases, including dementia, Alzheimer's, and other neurodegenerative conditions. It also plays a role in age-related cognitive decline, stroke, and Parkinson's disease.

One of the most effective ways to fight inflammation is through diet. Dining on foods rich in antioxidants, healthy fats, and whole grains, and avoiding foods that trigger inflammation, such as saturated and trans fats and refined carbs, help keep your brain in top shape. This way of eating, as exemplified in the Mediterranean diet, for example (▶13), has been shown to reduce the risk of Alzheimer's and vascular dementia. Another benefit: It can help you stay at a healthy weight. A 2009 study in the *Archives of Neurology* found that being obese in midlife increases the risk of developing dementia, possibly by double, according to some estimates. Another study in the journal *Neurology* confirmed that carrying more belly fat in middle age—a danger of declining midlife metabolism—also raises the risk of dementia down the road. If your BMI is over 30, try the tips in part II to lose weight and protect your brain.

Pile Produce on Your Plate for a Younger Brain

Fruits and vegetables are fantastic sources of antioxidants, vitamins, minerals, fiber, and other anti-inflammatory compounds called phytonutrients that help keep your brain young. Antioxidants fight free radicals that damage cells and trigger inflammation. Vitamins such as folate, found in broccoli, lentils and beans, spinach, and asparagus, help keep brain synapses firing correctly. And the thousands of phytonutrients in plant foods exert all kinds of beneficial brain effects, including mopping up free radicals. Color is one indication of which phytonutrients a plant contains, so eating a variety of brightly colored fruits and vegetables is the best way to ensure you get broad-spectrum protection against oxidative stress. Aim for five to nine servings a day.

Feast on Healthy Fats to Keep Your Brain in Top Shape

Omega-3s create hormones that dampen inflammation throughout your body—including your brain. They also thin your blood slightly, making it easier for your brain to get the oxygen-rich blood it needs to function optimally. A 2010 review of studies in *Current Alzheimer Research* noted that a higher intake of docosahexaenoic acid (DHA), one type of omega-3, is associated with a lower risk of Alzheimer's disease. Other research shows that a DHA deficit is linked to cognitive decline. Fatty, cold-water fish like wild salmon, lake trout, albacore tuna, herring, anchovies, and sardines are the best sources. Grass-fed beef, fortified foods (like eggs), walnuts, ground flaxseed, and soy foods like tofu contain omega-3s as well. And broccoli, cabbage, and other leafy greens supply small amounts. Choose wild-caught fish to reduce contaminants like mercury and PCBs that can harm brain health. The Monterey Bay Aquarium (montereybayaquarium.org) offers "Seafood Watch" guides for different parts of the United States, available online, that help you buy the best fish while protecting your health and the health of marine life. Experts recommend eating two servings of fatty fish or multiple servings of other omega-3-rich foods per week to benefit your brain.

Eat More Whole Grains to Slow Brain Aging

Whole grains contain fiber, which can scrub damaging plaques from your brain arteries. They also boast antioxidants and nutrients, like thiamin, that calm inflammation. Refined carbohydrates and sweets, on the other hand, spike your blood sugar and trigger inflammation. High blood sugar (anything over 100 mg/dL, the cutoff point for prediabetes) increases your risk of stroke. And research shows that excess insulin—produced in response to high blood sugar—accelerates brain aging and increases risk of cognitive impairment and dementia, including Alzheimer's disease. To keep your blood sugar steady, eat three servings of whole grains per day (half of your total grain intake). Your best bet is to eat actual whole grains, rather than whole-grain flours and products, which have been processed to remove some of the beneficial parts of the grain. Barley, oats (especially steel-cut), quinoa, millet, wheat berries, and brown rice are all good choices.

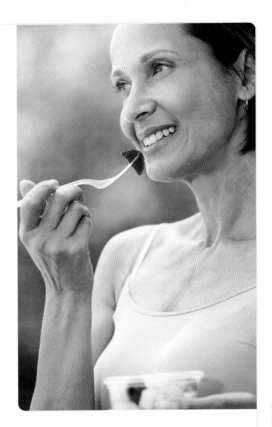

The Takeaway: Anti-Inflammatory Diet Basics

Eat five to nine servings of fruits and vegetables per day.

Eat two servings per week of fish high in omega-3 fats: wild salmon, albacore tuna, lake trout, sardines, or herring.

Eat three servings of whole grains per day.

26

Eat "Superfoods" to Stay Sharp As You Age

A few foods deserve to become dietary staples for their ability to boost memory, slow brain aging, and protect against cognitive decline. All these superfoods are stellar sources of antioxidants and have solid science behind their brain benefits. Antioxidants are critical for brain health because they fight free radicals, which can interfere with how your brain cells process nutrients, cause oxidative damage that can lead to cell death, and keep brain cells from communicating with each other, leading to memory loss. Make these antioxidant-rich foods a mealtime mainstay to mop up free radicals and keep your brain young.

Bet on Blueberries for Lifelong Brain Health

Blueberries contain a number of polyphenols, plant compounds that protect health. Of these, anthocyanins—water-soluble antioxidants that give fruits and vegetables a red or purple color—have shown particular benefit for the brain. In addition to their antioxidant and anti-inflammatory effects, anthocyanins may boost neuron signaling in brain centers associated with memory, as well as improve how the brain disposes of glucose, all of which may help prevent or slow memory decline. A 2010 study in the *Journal of Agricultural and Food Chemistry* found that older adults with mild memory problems who drank wild blueberry juice every day for twelve weeks showed improved scores on memory tests. Sprinkle a handful of blueberries on your oatmeal at breakfast, stir them into yogurt, swap your morning OJ for a glass of blueberry juice, or set out frozen berries for a cool summer dessert. Sugar wipes out anthocyanins, however, so don't rely on a slice of blueberry pie (or jam or muffins) for your daily dose.

Blackberries, raspberries, cherries, red grapes, pomegranates, red cabbage, and beets are also good sources of anthocyanins.

Cook with Curry for Clearer Thinking

Based on lab and animal studies, curcumin, the component of the curry spice turmeric responsible for its yellow color, appears to protect the brain in at least ten different ways. For example, it defends the brain against stress-induced memory problems, according to a 2009 study in the journal *Neuropharmacology*. Turkish researchers also showed that curcumin can help combat age-related cognitive decline stemming from elevated insulin levels (▶25). And a 2008 review of studies on the role of curcumin in Alzheimer's found that the spice improves memory by delaying the breakdown of neurons, decreasing plaque formation, removing toxic metals like cadmium and lead, calming inflammation, and fighting free radicals. Typical uses for turmeric include Indian curries, but you can also add a teaspoon to soups, rice dishes, sauces, and marinades, or even to scrambled eggs. Consuming turmeric along with black pepper significantly increases your body's ability to use curcumin (by up to 2,000 percent!), and healthy fats may enhance absorption as well.

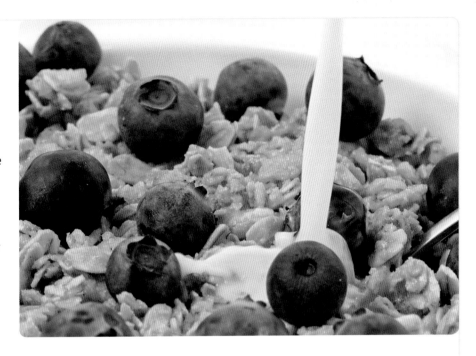

Pour an Occasional Glass to Protect Your Brain

Like blueberries, anthocyanins give red grapes their color. Purple grape juice and red wine are good sources, and vino also offers up another superstar antioxidant: resveratrol, found in the skins of grapes. Red wine contains higher concentrations of resveratrol than white wine (even though some varieties of white wine are made with red grapes) because it ferments with the skins longer during winemaking. Resveratrol boosts memory by limiting the breakdown of important neurotransmitters, according to a 2009 study in the *European Journal of Pharmacology*. And researchers at the Mount Sinai School of Medicine found that moderate red wine consumption helps prevent the formation of brain plaques in Alzheimer's, thereby reducing risk of the disease. Other studies confirm that resveratrol's antioxidant and anti-inflammatory activity protects the brain against age-related cognitive decline. Limit yourself to two glasses of red wine a week for women and three for men, though, since more can leach thiamin, a B vitamin that helps make necessary neurotransmitters and fights inflammation (▶**25**). Concord grape juice seems to be an equally healthy choice: A 2009 study in the *British Journal of Nutrition* found that the juice improved cognitive function in adults with early memory problems.

The Takeaway: Memory-Boosting Foods

Eat blueberries or drink blueberry juice every day.

Add a teaspoon of turmeric or curry powder to your scrambled eggs, rice, sauces, and other dishes. Add a dash of black pepper to increase your body's ability to use the spice.

Drink a glass of wine (two per week for women, three for men) or drink Concord grape juice to protect against Alzheimer's plaques and calm inflammation.

27

Exercise to Keep Your Brain Fit for Life

Studies show that exercise improves cognition by acting on both brain structure and function. For example, exercise builds brain tissue, according to a study at the University of Illinois. Researchers assigned groups of over-sixty adults to six months of either aerobic exercise or toning and stretching and found that aerobic exercisers had higher brain volume than the others, suggesting that exercise spares brain tissue lost during aging and enhances cognitive health.

A 2009 study in the journal *The Physician and Sportsmedicine* notes that exercise promotes the creation of new neurons, increases brain volume, and improves cognitive function—all of which help aging brains retain plasticity, or the ability to create new neural connections. Not only does exercise increase the number of neurons, but it also improves their

responsiveness and regulates important neurotransmitters responsible for cell communication, helping you stay sharp.

Regular exercise may also delay the onset of dementia and Alzheimer's disease, reported researchers in a 2006 study in the *Annals of Internal Medicine*. The study followed 1,740 people over the age of sixty-five and found that, over the course of six years, those who exercised at least three times a week were 32 percent less likely to be diagnosed with dementia during the study. The authors suggest that this reduced risk might be because frequent exercisers have less brain tissue loss in the hippocampus, one of the earliest areas of the brain to be affected by Alzheimer's disease.

Age-related damage to blood vessels and reduced blood flow to your brain (blood flow typically declines with age) can lead

to impaired mental function and even vascular dementia. So another advantage of exercise is that it boosts oxygen-rich blood flow to your brain. A small study in the *American Journal of Neuroradiology* revealed a possible reason for the increased circulation: Researchers found that, out of fourteen healthy adults in their sixties and seventies, those who exercised had more small blood vessels in their brains and less age-induced twisting in those vessels.

Exercise Daily to Delay Cognitive Decline

Experts aren't sure yet how long or hard you need to exercise for the best brain results, or if one type of exercise is better for your brain than others. But most recommend that you aim for at least thirty minutes of moderate aerobic exercise on most (or all) days of the week. In fact, a 2010 study published

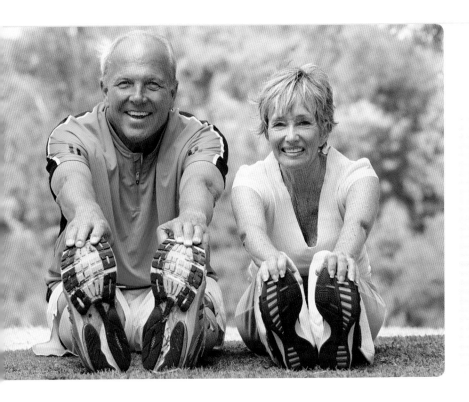

The Takeaway: Exercise Your Brain

Aim to exercise for thirty minutes on most days of the week, preferably outside.

Moderate exercise is better than light or vigorous exercise for cognitive health.

Strength training is just as important as aerobic exercise for keeping your brain in top shape.

in the *Archives of Neurology* found that moderate exercise in midlife or late life decreased the risk of mild cognitive impairment more than light or vigorous exercise. Exercising outdoors may boost brain health even more, suggests a 2008 study in the journal *Psychological Science*. Researchers found that people who walked in natural environments performed better on memory and attention tests than those exercising in urban settings.

Most research has focused on the benefits of aerobic exercise, but a 2010 study in the *Archives of Internal Medicine* demonstrated that strength training improves cognitive function as well. In the study, sixty-five- to seventy-five-year-old women who performed resistance training exercises (such as lunges and squats) once or twice a week had significantly better scores on tests measuring mental focus and conflict resolution than the control group, who did balance and toning exercises.

In addition to sustained exercise, daily activity may also help you keep your wits about you. In a 2008 study in the *Journal of the American Geriatrics Society*, researchers asked more than 2,700 women in their eighties to wear a watchlike device that measured all of their daytime movement, from walking to gardening to shopping to playing bridge. The women who were the most active showed better cognitive function and were the least likely to show signs of cognitive impairment.

In short, the same kinds of activity that benefit the rest of your body are good for your brain as well. The most important thing is that you get moving!

28

Keep Chronic Illness at Bay to Boost Brain Health

You may be surprised to find that underlying health problems can make it harder to remember someone's name or puzzle through a complex problem. But research has consistently linked high blood pressure, diabetes, and obesity (▶25) to an increased risk of cognitive decline. Preventing or controlling those chronic conditions now may not only protect you from serious problems like Alzheimer's down the road, but it may even help you think more clearly today.

Get a Handle on High Blood Pressure to Keep Your Brain Healthy

You know that having high blood pressure puts you at risk for heart disease, but increasing evidence shows it can also affect your brain health. Two large, recent studies show a significant link between high blood pressure and the risk of dementia, including Alzheimer's disease. High blood pressure, or hypertension, can damage tiny blood vessels in the brain and lead to scarring (called lesions) in the brain's white matter, its communication system. That breakdown in brain cell communication leads to cognitive decline and dementia. In both studies, systolic blood pressure (the top number) was the critical factor, and since the damage was cumulative, the researchers emphasized that getting and keeping blood pressure under control in early and midlife is essential to protect your brain as you get older.

The first study, published in 2009 in the *Journal of Clinical Hypertension*, looked at brain scans of more than 1,400 postmenopausal women and found that those who had blood pressure above 140/90 mm Hg (hypertension)—whether or not they were taking blood pressure medication—had more and larger white matter lesions than those whose blood pressure was under control. The second study, published in 2010 in the journal *Stroke*, found that white matter damage increased with every twenty-point jump in systolic blood pressure.

Getting your blood pressure down to 120/80 mm Hg or below not only appears to protect you against dementia, but it also significantly lowers your risk of stroke and other blood vessel damage. The National Institutes of Health is currently investigating whether aggressively treating hypertension to lower systolic blood pressure to below 120 ("normal") offers additional health benefits. This Systolic Blood Pressure Intervention Trial (SPRINT) study is the first clinical trial of its kind and is expected to have results by 2018. Until then, talk to your doctor about how lifestyle changes and supplements can keep your blood pressure under control (▶ **52**), or whether or not you should take medication.

Avoid Diabetes to Preserve Cognition

Experts are still trying to figure out exactly how diabetes influences brain health, but research shows that diabetics are one-and-a-half times more likely to experience mild cognitive impairment, vascular dementia, and Alzheimer's disease than people without diabetes. High blood sugar, excess insulin, and problems with insulin sensitivity all appear to be factors (▶ **25**), affecting brain cells, memory function, and your ability to learn. For example, a 2009 study in the journal *Diabetes Care* found that even a 1 percent increase in A1C levels (a long-term measure of blood sugar) was linked to lower scores on cognitive tests. Other research reveals that people with and without diabetes who have poor blood sugar control—either too high or too low—have worse cognitive performance.

Insulin is also critical for good brain health: It helps transport glucose to brain cells for energy and plays a role in many brain functions, including cognitive processes. When your brain doesn't have enough insulin, or if the insulin isn't working properly (called insulin resistance), it can result in cognitive decline. Insulin resistance, for example, seems to be a factor in Alzheimer's, since people with the disease can't regulate their blood sugar as efficiently. And studies show that too much insulin can age your brain and increase risk of cognitive decline and dementia, including Alzheimer's disease.

To protect your brain, as well as the rest of your body, aim to keep your blood sugar under 100 mg/dL, the cutoff point for prediabetes. Exercising regularly and eating fewer processed and refined foods will go a long way toward preventing or controlling diabetes (▶ **13, 25, 50, 55**). And if you already have diabetes, your best bet for brain health is to work with your doctor to keep tight control over your blood sugar levels.

The Takeaway: Chronic Health, Not Illness

Rely on lifestyle changes or take medication to lower your high blood pressure.

Exercise regularly and eat fewer processed foods to reduce the risk of diabetes.

If you have diabetes, keep tight control over your blood sugar levels.

29

Set Up a Strong Social Support System to Prevent Cognitive Decline

As you get older, your natural points of connection with others change and often diminish. Whether from retirement, a newly empty nest, or loved ones moving or passing away, you may find that the support structure you once had in place is smaller and looks much different than it used to. Health issues may also force you—or your friends or family—to cut back on certain activities, curtailing your connections to others. If you don't take steps to maintain existing relationships and create new ones, a sense of isolation can creep in, bringing with it a higher risk of depression and cognitive decline.

The second half of life brings with it opportunities to deepen friendships and expand your social circle. Plenty of research shows the brain benefits of a strong social network. For example, a landmark MacArthur Foundation study published in 1999 found that maintaining social and intellectual connections was one of the most significant characteristics of successful aging among the more than one thousand adults who participated in the study. A 2008 study in the *American Journal of Public Health* suggested that larger social networks protect cognitive function. And having an active social life is one important factor, along with mental and physical activity, in improving cognition and protecting against dementia, according to a 2004 study in *Lancet Neurology*. A later study in the same journal noted that people with larger social networks had higher cognitive function in Alzheimer's, especially in the areas of working memory (remembering recently learned information) and semantic memory (language-based ability to recall words and facts).

So what does it mean to have a strong social network? The number, frequency, and degree of interactions with others all factor in, and all kinds of links—from waving at a neighbor to sharing deep concerns with a trusted friend—are included. "Having that social network, however it is built, is what is important," says Sarah Lovegreen, M.P.H., a health manager with OASIS, a national organization that promotes lifelong learning and service for adults age fifty and older.

Make New Friends, but Keep the Old

In addition to strengthening existing relationships, you can stay socially engaged and help your brain by meeting and befriending new people. In fact, meeting people can forge new neural connections, and interacting with others activates several areas of your brain.

To find new friends, it helps to open yourself up to novel experiences. Join a book club, take a cooking class, sign up for a group travel experience, or even gather a few acquaintances for a friendly debate about a topic of common interest (brain bonus: You'll have to think on your feet and express yourself clearly). If you find new experiences intimidating and meeting new people exhausting, enlist a friend to join you. Having that base of connection can make it easier to step out of your comfort zone and introduce yourself to unfamiliar people and situations.

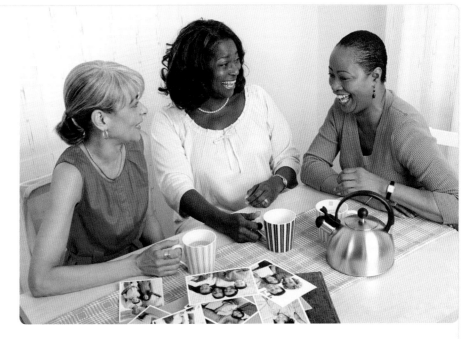

Volunteering is a great way to keep engaged in your community and meet new people, and it can provide a sense of purpose. Ask about opportunities at your library, museums, hospitals, community centers, schools, or a house of worship. If you're caring for an ailing family member, consider joining a support group to get to know people in similar circumstances and learn new ways of coping.

Instead of plopping down on the couch to watch another episode of *Law & Order*, break out of your rut and invite your spouse or a friend for a walk. In fact, combining social and physical activity gives you even better brain benefits, notes Lovegreen. Walking or running clubs, exercise classes, group hikes, or playing a few rounds of golf with friends are all excellent ways to get fit and expand your social circle at the same time.

Combining social and intellectual pursuits is another way to meet people and stay sharp (remember the MacArthur study, p. 74). Start a chess club, attend a lecture, teach a class, or volunteer to tutor in your local schools. In addition to forming friendships, you may discover a new passion—all while boosting your brainpower and protecting against cognitive decline.

The Takeaway: Social Connections

Continue to make new friends through volunteering, taking a class, or joining a group.

Combine social interaction with physical exercise or intellectual activities to multiply their benefits.

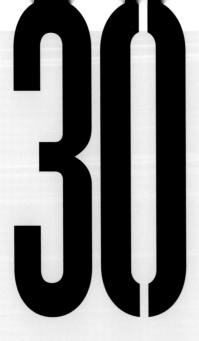

30

Defeat Depression and Stress to Minimize Brain Aging

Research shows that cognitive functions like learning, memory, and higher-level thinking and decision making take a considerable hit as you get older. The areas of the brain responsible for those functions—the medial temporal lobe (hippocampus) and prefrontal cortex—are also susceptible to depression and stress, which can amplify age-related cognitive decline. Thankfully, you can keep your brain young and healthy by adopting lifestyle changes that protect against depression and stress.

Prevent or Conquer Depression to Think Clearly for Years to Come

People in late life are more prone to depression, which can cause stress, trigger pain, aggravate chronic conditions, and age your brain. Evidence, including a 2010 study in the journal *Psychiatry Research*, suggests that major depressive disorder can have harmful

and lasting effects on cognitive function. A 2010 study in the *British Journal of Psychiatry* did brain scans on people over the age of sixty who had major depression and found that cognitive deficits due to depression most likely stem from blood vessel damage in the brain (the scarring results in white matter lesions [▶28]). Depression especially affects your ability to understand language and process information quickly, making you feel fuzzy-headed, according to a 2010 study in *Neuropsychobiology*. And mild depression can trigger brain changes as well, so even if you're just feeling a little blue, it's worth taking steps to deal with the depression before it does too much damage.

Whether you are depressed, think you might be, or are concerned about keeping depression at bay as you get older, your first step is to talk to your doctor about

lifestyle changes that can protect against depression and even help lift it. For example, countless studies demonstrate exercise's ability to stimulate endorphins, those feel-good neurotransmitters, and boost mood. A 2006 study by Canadian researchers suggests that exercise might also alleviate depression by stimulating new neurons. Exercise can help you hang on to functional ability longer as well, allowing you to stay active, live independently, and maintain social connections—all of which can help you ward off depression. "Staying socially engaged, whether that's going to church or taking a class, is one of the best tools to combat depression," notes Sarah Lovegreen, M.P.H., health manager with OASIS, a national organization that promotes lifelong learning and service for adults age fifty and older. "We're social creatures…we don't live in isolation." (▶29)

If these strategies don't suffice, talk to your doctor about medications that might help. Be sure to discuss potential side effects (▸73), since those can significantly affect your quality of life.

Stop Stress in Its Tracks for Lifelong Brainpower

Moderate amounts of stress hormones can actually improve cognitive function and memory, but exposing your brain to too much for too long can mess with your mind. The hippocampus, the area of your brain responsible for long-term memory and spatial navigation, has more glucocorticoid receptors (for stress hormones, such as cortisol) than other parts of the brain, making it more vulnerable to chronic stress. As you get older, your hippocampus undergoes changes—such as losing synapses and having them become less responsive—and adding stress to the picture accelerates that brain aging, affecting memory and your speed of processing information. Stress hormones may also kill brain cells and shrink your hippocampus.

But keeping anxiety in check appears to undo stress-related damage and helps keep your brain working at its best. A 2010 study in the *Journal of Neuroscience* noted that counteracting cortisol restores spatial memory, keeps synapses adaptable to taking in new experiences (called plasticity, which is the basis for learning and memory and typically declines with age), and helps neurons in your hippocampus fire properly.

Simple strategies (▸18, 56, 61, 85, 97) can help you subdue stress and "get your brain back." As with depression, having friends to turn to in difficult times is key. Take a deep breath, or try breathing exercises (▸4); people often breathe shallowly when stressed, and lack of oxygen for the brain can affect your memory and damage your hippocampus. And try keeping a calendar or to-do list to stay focused: Decision making and planning are use-it-or-lose-it components of cognitive health, and having a plan for the day can help you feel more in control.

The Takeaway: Beat Depression and Stress

Exercise to lift your mood; even ten minutes can relieve the blues.

Stay socially connected; isolation worsens depression, which results in foggy thinking.

Reduce stress by taking deep breaths.

Keep a calendar and lists to manage your busy life and help you make decisions.

31

Increase Your Mental Focus with Mind-Body Techniques

Feeling scattered and easily distracted, forgetting items on your to-do list or the names of people you've just met, walking into a room with no memory of why you went there in the first place—these are some of the most common, and annoying, aspects of brain aging and the resulting cognitive decline. But certain mind-body practices can help you regain focus and stay sharp as you get older. More than just memory tricks, these techniques can actually change neural pathways and strengthen your mental muscle. Put them into practice now to reap immediate brain benefits; they're even more effective the longer you do them.

Meditate to Maintain Your Mental Acuity

Although researchers aren't sure yet just how meditation protects against age-related cognitive decline and dementia, mounting evidence suggests it can slow brain aging in a number of ways. For example, meditation can relieve memory-sapping stress (▶ 30) and prevent oxidative damage from free radicals (▶ 26), and it may also strengthen brain cell circuits and communication and offset age-related shrinking of your brain's cerebral cortex (the area that controls memory, language, and sensory processing).

In broad terms, there are two main forms of meditation: focused attention and open monitoring. Focused attention meditation means concentrating on an object, a word, your breath, or another element for a sustained period. Open monitoring, or mindfulness meditation, involves being present in the moment to evaluate experiences without reacting to or judging them, helping you to recognize patterns of emotion and thought.

A 2006 study in *Nature Neuroscience* found that lapses in attention result from reduced activity in the parts of your brain responsible for concentration, which leads to less efficient processing of the situation at hand. However, researchers noted in a 2008 review of studies that several aspects of attention can be learned, such as detecting and disengaging from distraction and redirecting your attention back to your original point of focus. They concluded that focused attention meditation can help you hone those skills. Research also shows that this type of meditation can boost blood flow to the brain, bringing oxygen and glucose needed for energy and optimal functioning.

Open monitoring meditation may help synchronize neuron firing, an important feature of synapse "plasticity" (or adaptability), which is the basis for learning and memory, and typically declines with age. It can also help increase your ability to focus.

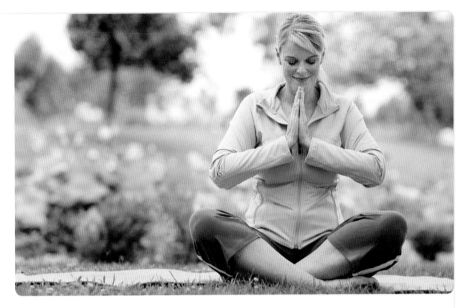

More studies are needed to determine which kind of meditation has the biggest brain benefits, whether there are important common elements in the different kinds, and what "dose" you need to reap the most mental gains, but as little as ten minutes a day can make a difference. Working up to thirty to forty minutes a day may bring additional benefits. Perhaps the most common types are Transcendental Meditation (a form of focused attention meditation using a mantra) and mindfulness meditation (open monitoring, involving being mindful of your surroundings or experience). The Mayo Clinic offers information about different forms of meditation and suggestions for trying them at www .mayoclinic.com/health/meditation /HQ01070. Most forms involve sitting still in a quiet place, but if you find it difficult to quiet your thoughts while staying stationary, try a walking meditation (brain bonus: exercise! [▶27]).

Use Mind-Body Approaches to Relax and Retrain Your Brain

Yoga, guided imagery, prayer, and progressive muscle relaxation are other mind-body techniques you can use to boost brain health. Their main benefit is stress reduction (▶30), but they offer other mental advantages as well. Yoga, for instance, also increases circulation to bring oxygen-rich blood to the brain. Guided imagery—forming mental pictures about relaxing places or situations—stimulates your imagination and senses, and a 2004 study in *Psychological Reports* indicates that it can also improve working memory (responsible for helping you hold on to recently learned bits of information). Other research on guided imagery suggests that being more relaxed can help you process information better. Prayer shares similarities with meditation, and a 2009 study in the *Journals of Gerontology: Biological Sciences and Medical Sciences* further noted that regularly attending religious services is associated with a lower risk of cognitive decline. Finally, progressive muscle relaxation, which involves slowly tightening and relaxing muscles starting at your toes or head and moving up or down the body, respectively, helps you let go of tension in your body and mind, preparing you to learn and remember information more easily.

The Takeaway: Mind-Body Relaxation

Meditate for ten minutes a day, working up to thirty minutes.

Do yoga or a walking meditation to reap the combined mental benefits of stress reduction and exercise.

Pray and regularly attend religious services to reduce cognitive decline.

32

Snooze Your Way to a Younger Brain

You probably don't need a study to tell you that not getting enough sleep can make it hard to think clearly and remember things. But research does show that sleep deprivation can affect cognition, and since your sleep patterns change and your risk of sleep problems increases as you get older (▶19), not getting enough shut-eye can aggravate age-related cognitive decline. A 2009 study by Israeli researchers found that older adults with chronic insomnia (a common late-life complaint) scored much worse on cognitive tests measuring memory span, attention, time estimation, working memory (retaining recently learned information), and integration of two dimensions than those without sleep complaints. Ultimately, the researchers suggested, improving sleep may help maintain cognitive function in older adults.

Sleep is critical for memory formation and recall because it consolidates and encodes memories in your brain to make them easier to retrieve when you're awake. Declarative memories (facts, or things you consciously remember and can explain in words) are most affected by slow wave sleep, the first stage of deep sleep. Rapid eye movement (REM) sleep is the second stage of deep sleep, when dreams generally occur, and it benefits procedural (skill-based) and emotional memory. And while mental fatigue is obvious after an all-nighter, research shows that gradually accumulating a sleep debt might even be more harmful because you're less likely to notice the resulting cognitive decline. A 2003 study in the journal *Sleep* found that people who consistently got six or fewer hours of sleep per night for two weeks scored just as poorly on cognitive tests as those who experienced two nights of total

sleep deprivation. What's more, after a few nights of limited sleep, the volunteers didn't feel sleepier during the day or realize that their cognitive performance was gradually getting worse. The takeaway, researchers wrote, is that "even relatively moderate sleep restriction can seriously impair waking neurobehavioral functions in healthy adults."

Another sneaky brain-sapping side effect of sleep deprivation is its link to depression (▶30). Older adults are more likely to experience both depression and sleep problems, and while researchers aren't sure if depression leads to sleep problems or vice versa, they acknowledge it's easy to sink into a self-perpetuating cycle of the two. Conversely, improving sleep or treating depression can benefit both conditions and lead to better brain function.

Get More Zzzs to Keep Your Brain in Top Shape

If you have a chronic sleep problem, like insomnia, restless legs syndrome, or obstructive sleep apnea (all of which are more common as you get older), talk to your doctor or a sleep specialist to design a treatment plan. Certain health conditions or medications may trigger sleep problems as well; work with your doctor to get health issues under control or switch medicines if needed.

If health problems aren't interfering with your sleep, there are some easy ways to ensure a good night's rest. Start by determining how much sleep you actually need (most people over fifty require between seven and nine hours a night). Try going to bed at a consistent time and letting yourself wake up naturally without an alarm for a full week, without napping during the day if possible. At the end of the week, in theory, you will have made up for a good portion of your sleep debt and should be able to determine your nighttime sleep needs. Once you know how much you need, you may find you have to alter your bedtime routine in order to get the full amount. Lifestyle changes like setting a regular sleep schedule and keeping your bedroom dark can help you fall and stay asleep (▶ 19, 63). If you need help getting drowsy for an earlier bedtime, about an hour beforehand dim the lights and switch to quieter activities, like reading a lighthearted book or meditating. Taking a hot bath or shower before bed also helps by raising your core body temperature—once you're out of the hot water, the resulting temperature drop allows you to fall asleep faster and sleep more soundly. Avoid drinking alcohol or consuming caffeine for three to four hours before bed, and if you still have trouble sleeping, cut them out completely. If an overactive mind is keeping you awake, stash a notebook on your nightstand to write down concerns or tomorrow's to-do list and try a mind-body technique like progressive muscle relaxation (▶ 31) to help quiet your mind. If you've tried all these lifestyle changes and are still having trouble sleeping, consider taking melatonin or another natural remedy (▶ 63). Prescription sleep aids can also be effective, but they carry greater risks of potentially serious side effects and may be habit-forming—use them as a last resort.

The Takeaway: Sweet Dreams

To figure out how much sleep you need (probably between seven and nine hours), go to bed and wake up without an alarm for a week, and don't nap during the day.

To help you nod off, dim the lights an hour before bedtime and transition to quiet activities like reading a book or meditating.

Take a hot shower or bath before bed; the drop in your body temperature afterward will help you fall asleep.

33

Stimulate Your Brain to Improve Cognition As You Get Older

Your brain circuitry is not hardwired—it's actually quite adaptable. The scientific term is plasticity, and although it decreases with age, your adult brain retains a significant capacity to modify itself based on your experiences and how you interact with your environment. Plasticity is considered the basis for learning and memory, and losing it can lead to age-related cognitive decline. But consistently challenging your brain and exposing yourself to new people, places, and experiences can form new brain cells, strengthen neural connections so you can store and retrieve information more easily, and keep your brain young.

Break Out of a Rut to Grow New Brain Cells

Studies show that novelty boosts neural responses. That means doing the same job, and the same hobbies, in the same routine doesn't necessarily count toward keeping you cognitively active. "If you're at work doing the same ten activities, is that really cognitively stimulating? Those activities are already programmed," notes Sarah Lovegreen, M.P.H., health manager with OASIS, a national organization that promotes lifelong learning and service for adults age fifty and older. "So challenging your mind to learn a new skill, think in a new way, challenge opinions, or expose you to new ideas is more effective."

One way to work novelty into your life is through leisure activities. In one *New England Journal of Medicine* study, people over seventy-five who participated in hobbies such as reading, playing board games, playing musical instruments, and dancing reduced their risk of dementia. For the best brain benefits, try something you haven't done before, or at least attempt a variation on the theme. If you enjoy swing dancing, give the tango a twirl. Loved learning French? Challenge yourself to pick up Spanish or Italian. If you play the piano, put down classical music for a while and try your hand at jazz or blues.

Changing your environment can also engage your brain by challenging your visual and spatial memory and stimulating your senses. It can be as dramatic as rearranging your furniture and painting your walls a new color, or as minor as organizing your drawers differently and growing some fragrant herbs. You can also try taking a new route to familiar places like the grocery store.

Go Beyond Crossword Puzzles to Boost Your Brainpower

Crosswords, Sudoku, and other puzzles and memory exercises can be mentally stimulating, and research shows they're

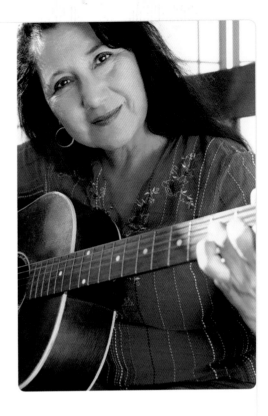

great additions to your brain-boosting toolkit. A 2002 study in the *Journal of the American Medical Association* followed a group of eight hundred adults over the age of sixty-five to see how participating in stimulating activities protected cognitive function. They found that people who did activities that involved processing information—such as watching TV; listening to the radio; reading newspapers, magazines, and books; playing games such as cards, checkers, crosswords, or other puzzles; and going to museums—nearly every day reduced their risk of developing Alzheimer's disease by almost 50 percent. And the more cognitively active they were, the less decline they experienced in global cognition (by 47 percent), working memory (by 60 percent), and perceptual speed (by 30 percent), compared to those who rarely or never engaged in stimulating behaviors.

You can also use technology to challenge your brain. For example, a 2009 study in the *American Journal of Geriatric Psychiatry* found that searching the Internet increases brain activity, especially in the areas of decision making and complex reasoning. And the Wii and Nintendo DS game systems offer brain-teasing games that provide mental stimulation while forcing you to learn how to use the interface.

As powerfully protective as these activities are, however, they don't offer social connection or physical activity, two other important tenets of brain health. You'll have an even better brain benefit if you can combine some aspects of intellectual, physical, and social stimulation, notes Lovegreen. If you'd like to learn knitting, see if a local yarn shop or craft store offers group classes. Interested in genetic research at the zoo? Ask if the staff offers lectures or other public programs. If you love to read, see if a local bookstore holds author signings or discussion groups. Or invite a friend to explore a walking or hiking path in a different neighborhood or to take skating lessons with you.

The Takeaway: Brain Boosters

Do something different in your daily routine: Take a new route home, try a twist on your hobby, or rearrange the furniture.

Use technology, which is always changing, to stimulate your brain. Search the Web, or play a video game.

Combine mentally stimulating activities with social interactions or exercise to double the brain benefits.

34

Avoid These Brain Agers

As you might suspect, certain substances wreak havoc with your brain, and you should avoid them at all cost. Illicit drugs like marijuana increase paranoia and psychosis, and cocaine puts you at great risk for stroke and may also raise your risk of Parkinson's disease. Even legal drugs like nicotine can restrict blood flow to the brain, damaging it and causing premature aging. But not all brain agers are that clear-cut. For example, while small amounts of caffeine can increase alertness and even boost mental performance, downing too much can also restrict blood flow to the brain and interfere with much-needed sleep (▶32). And even though some types of dietary fat and alcohol can provide brain benefits (▶25, 26), the wrong kinds or excessive amounts can negatively affect your cognitive health over time if you're not careful.

Shun Saturated and Trans Fats to Stay Sharp As You Age

Emerging research links saturated and trans fats to an increased risk of age-related cognitive decline and dementia, including Alzheimer's disease, although researchers aren't sure exactly how they raise your risk. Saturated and trans fats trigger inflammation in the brain and actually prevent healthy fats like monounsaturated and omega-3 fatty acids from entering your brain cells. Additionally, a 2009 study in the journal *Progress in Lipid Research* suggested that regularly eating too much saturated fat and cholesterol disrupts the blood-brain barrier, allowing plasma proteins like amyloid-beta (sticky substances that clump together to form plaques typical in Alzheimer's disease) to leak into the brain and accumulate. A large 2006 study by Swedish researchers followed a group of nearly 1,500 people

for twenty years and found that even a moderate intake of saturated fat at midlife increased risk of dementia and Alzheimer's. For the best brain health, get less than 7 percent of your daily calories from saturated fat. An anti-inflammatory diet (▶25) is a smart choice because it limits foods high in saturated fat and cholesterol (animal products like meat and full-fat dairy).

Trans fats, or partially hydrogenated oils, undergo a chemical process to make them stable and solid at room temperature. Like other fats, they get incorporated into your cell membranes, but trans fats make your brain cells hard and rigid, slowing mental response time and accelerating brain aging. Trans fats are primarily found in commercial baked goods (cookies, cakes, chips, crackers, etc.) and fried foods like doughnuts and french fries. Thanks to a sneaky loophole, food products in the United States are allowed to claim they have 0 gram of trans fats when they contain less than 0.5 gram per serving. That may not seem like much, but those little bits can add up quickly. Instead of looking at the nutrition facts label, you'll need to examine the ingredients list. If you see the word shortening or partially hydrogenated anything, put the package back on the shelf.

Imbibe Moderately for Long-Term Brain Health

Yes, a glass of red wine can provide brain-protecting antioxidants and calm inflammation (▶ **26**), but overdoing it can deplete levels of glutathione (the brain's primary antioxidant) and thiamin (a B vitamin critical for brain function) and dehydrate you. A 2007 study in the *Journal of the American College of Nutrition* noted that being dehydrated can also cloud cognitive performance.

Not surprisingly, continually drinking too much can lead to alcohol-related brain damage. Heavy drinking also interferes with your brain's ability to process and use docosahexaenoic acid (DHA), a type of omega-3 vital for brain health (▶ **25**). And Australian researchers identified a history of harmful alcohol consumption as one of the biggest risk factors for cognitive impairment in older people.

But research shows that even moderate drinking may cause your brain to shrink over time and lead to abnormalities in how your brain transports glucose, oxygen, and other substances. The effect is more noticeable in women, possibly because they are smaller. To set yourself up for the best brain health in late life, limit your intake to no more than one drink a day (even better, two drinks a week for women and three for men), and be sure to drink a glass of water for each alcoholic beverage you imbibe to stay hydrated. You may also want to nix the nightcap: Alcohol can interfere with the deepest levels of sleep and cause you to wake up frequently, leading to daytime sleepiness and decreased cognitive function (▶ **32**).

The Takeaway: Brain Agers

Stay away from illegal drugs like marijuana and cocaine, which can result in pathologies ranging from paranoia to Parkinson's.

Limit your use of legal drugs like caffeine and nicotine, which restrict blood flow to the brain and can interfere with sleep.

Reduce your consumption of saturated fat (less than 7 percent of daily calories) and trans fats (as little as possible).

Don't drink more than one alcoholic beverage a day; preferably limit intake to two per week for women and three per week for men.

35

Clean Up Your Environment to Slow Brain Aging

Environmental toxins cause trouble for your brain in a number of ways; creating free radicals and increasing brain-aging inflammation are among them. Your body has an efficient detoxification system and can eliminate many of the toxic health threats you face every day. But since experts aren't sure how chronic, low-level exposure to the thousands of chemicals in our everyday environment interact with each other to affect us long-term, it makes sense to reduce your exposure—especially to known brain agers—whenever you can.

Avoid BPA and Other Endocrine Disruptors to Delay Mental Decline

Estrogen and testosterone appear to play critical roles in cognition and mood by affecting synapse "plasticity," which influences learning and memory and typically decreases with age. Endocrine disruptors like bisphenol A (BPA) and phthalates upset the delicate balance of hormones needed for your brain to work at its best. Combined with a natural decrease in sex hormones as you get older, studies suggest exposure to even low doses of endocrine disruptors may have widespread effects on brain structure and function, potentially speeding up age-related cognitive decline.

BPA is a synthetic substance used to create polycarbonate plastics, widely used in water bottles, food storage containers, and the lining of metal food cans, among other things. Research shows that it can leach into food and drinks, and that we are widely exposed to low, but continuous, levels. Most of the studies on BPA have been done on animals—usually rats—so researchers can't say for sure that the effects are the same in humans. But a 2008 study by Yale University researchers found that administering BPA to monkeys at a daily dose equal to the current U.S. Environmental Protection Agency's reference safe daily limit (50 micrograms per kilogram of body weight) interfered with synapse formation in the hippocampus and prefrontal cortex, two areas of the brain critical for cognition, attention, and memory. Phthalates hinder testosterone's effects on the brain, and a 2009 study in the *Journal of Applied Toxicology* found that low levels decreased spatial learning and reference memory in male rats.

With this mounting evidence, experts agree your best bet is to avoid endocrine disruptors as much as possible to preserve brain health and function as you get older. Many manufacturers are phasing out BPA—most notably makers of baby bottles and water bottles—and will often state on the label that a product is "BPA-free." Phthalates are frequently found in food packaging and plastic wrap, as well as personal care products like moisturizers, perfumes, hairsprays, soaps, and shampoos. You can reduce your exposure to these endocrine disruptors by using metal, glass, ceramic, or wooden products instead of plastic whenever possible, such as switching to glass or ceramic food storage containers. Also, avoid heating plastic containers in the microwave or running them through the dishwasher. Read the labels on personal care products and avoid those that list phthalates. Products that note "fragrance" on the label may include phthalates, even if they're not listed specifically. To research a particular product, check the Environmental Working Group website (www.ewg .org), which features a database of cosmetics ingredients.

Pare Down Your Pesticide Exposure to Preserve Brain Health

Chemical pesticides kill pests by attacking delicate nerve tissue. While they're designed to be safe for humans in small doses, the residue gets stored in your fat cells and can stay in your body indefinitely. Over time, levels build up and can raise your risk of Parkinson's and other neurological diseases. A 2008 study in the journal *Chemico-Biological Interactions* noted that chronic low-dose exposure to organophosphorus pesticides (the most commonly used

class of pesticides in the United States) results in cognitive impairment. Pesticides can also age your brain by triggering inflammation and increasing damaging free radicals.

To limit your contact, avoid using chemical pesticides in and around your home (*Organic Gardening* magazine, online at www.organicgardening.com, has suggestions for effective natural pest control methods) and eat organic produce whenever you can. If you don't have access to many organic foods or can't afford to eat entirely organic, the Environmental Working Group website www.foodnews.org provides a list of the fruits and vegetables that have the most pesticide residue to help you figure out where you'll get the most bang for your buck.

The Takeaway: Avoid Toxins

Look for water bottles and food storage containers that are "BPA-free"—or better yet, use glass, ceramic, or wooden containers. Don't run plastic food containers or bottles through the dishwasher.

Another toxic endocrine disruptor, phthalates, can be found in plastic wraps and personal care products; don't microwave plastic wrap or food packaging, and check product labels to avoid this memory-reducing chemical.

Reduce your exposure to pesticides by eating organic produce and using natural pest control methods.

36

Use Supplements and Drugs to Keep Your Brain Healthy for a Lifetime

While researchers are actively studying supplements and prescription and over-the-counter drugs to fight age-related cognitive decline, Alzheimer's, and Parkinson's disease, there isn't actually a lot of evidence to say what a healthy, middle-aged person should take to boost brain health and stave off future problems. What's more, the studies that do exist frequently contradict each other, leaving even the experts scratching their heads. As science continues to search for the brain-health magic bullet, here are some of the best-researched options that may protect your brain and help you stay sharp.

Arm Yourself with Antioxidants to Age Healthfully

Growing research suggests that cognitive decline and age-related diseases like Alzheimer's result from free-radical damage in the brain. While few studies have shown consistent results from individual supplements, antioxidants like vitamins C and E are proven free-radical fighters and work synergistically to protect cells from oxidative damage. Because vitamin E is fat soluble, it has access to parts of the brain (which is more than 60 percent fat) that other antioxidants can't reach, making it especially valuable. A 2004 study in the journal *Archives of Neurology* found that older adults who took 500 milligrams of vitamin C and 400 IU of vitamin E supplements together had lower risk of developing Alzheimer's disease. If you supplement with vitamin E, look for mixed natural tocopherols or d-alpha tocopherol rather than the synthetic form, dl-alpha tocopherol.

Coenzyme Q10 (CoQ10) is another fat-soluble antioxidant able to get into fatty brain cell membranes and protect them from free radicals. It's made by every cell in your body and helps the mitochondria—cell structures responsible for producing energy—do their job. With aging, however, levels of CoQ10 decline, and your brain may not have enough to perform all of its critical functions or to protect itself against free radicals. Preliminary studies show encouraging results with supplementing for Alzheimer's and especially Parkinson's disease, but more research in humans is needed. For basic brain health, start with 30 milligrams a day.

Give Ginkgo a Try for Clearer Thinking

Ginkgo biloba is possibly the best-known supplement for brain health, but research shows mixed results. Ginkgo contains antioxidant compounds called flavonoids and terpenoids that can help prevent free-radical damage to the brain that might impair mental function. It also increases blood flow to the brain, potentially enhancing memory. There is plenty of promising research on the herb not just for preventing cognitive decline but also for improving existing dementia and Alzheimer's. For example, a 2010 review of studies in the journal *Pharmacopsychiatry* found that using standardized ginkgo biloba extract for six months improved cognitive function in people with dementia. And a 2009 review of studies in *Human Psychopharmacology* noted that consistently taking ginkgo improves higher-level thinking and long-term memory.

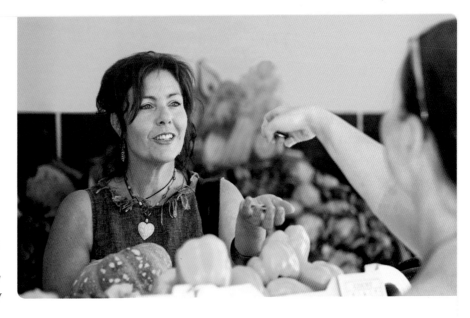

However, two large, long-term studies published recently in the *Journal of the American Medical Association* found that ginkgo biloba did not reduce cognitive decline or prevent dementia in people taking 120 milligrams twice a day. The researchers acknowledged that more than 40 percent of the subjects dropped out of the study before it ended (a definite drawback), and participants were all more than seventy years old, so starting the supplement earlier in life may still protect brain function. Ginkgo is safe and relatively inexpensive, so if you'd like to try it, take 120 milligrams once or twice a day (the amount used in most studies).

Mind Your Medications for Mental Longevity

Some studies show that nonsteroidal anti-inflammatory drugs (NSAIDs), such as ibuprofen or naproxen, may prevent Alzheimer's. A 2008 study in *Alzheimer's* & *Dementia* found that people with the Apo E-4 gene (a marker of increased risk for Alzheimer's) who took a combination of NSAIDs, 500 milligrams of vitamin C, and 400 IU of vitamin E at least four times a week showed less cognitive decline than nonusers. Taking NSAIDs regularly may raise homocysteine levels, which can aggravate neurological problems such as inflammation, depression, memory problems, and cognitive decline; take a vitamin B-50 complex supplement to keep levels in check. NSAIDs have some side effects, in particular gastrointestinal problems and the possibility of rebound headaches, so ask your doctor if the risks outweigh the benefits for you.

Although early research on statins, which are normally used for lowering cholesterol, proved promising for also preventing dementia, later studies have failed to show any benefit. Statins also significantly slow your ability to produce brain-boosting CoQ10 (▶ **59**), so if

▶ **59** you take statins for cholesterol, add a 50-milligram CoQ10 supplement to your regimen.

The Takeaway: Supplements and Drugs for Brain Health

Take 500 milligrams of vitamin C and 400 IU of vitamin E supplements daily (and ask your doctor about adding an NSAID four times a week). With vitamin E, look for mixed natural tocopherols or d-alpha tocopherol rather than the synthetic form, dl-alpha tocopherol.

Take coenzyme Q10 (CoQ10) to fight free radicals in the brain.

Try 120 milligrams of ginkgo biloba once or twice a day to preserve, and possibly improve, long-term memory and cognitive function.

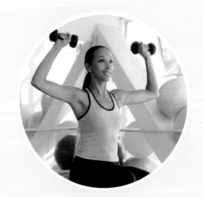
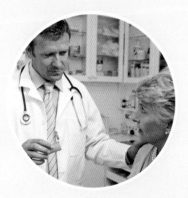
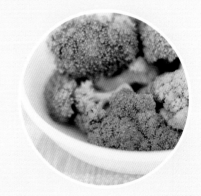
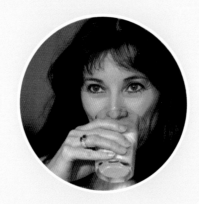
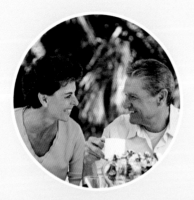
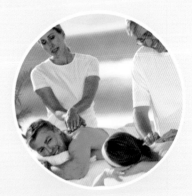

PART IV

Turn Back the Clock on Your
Bones and Joints

37

Assess Your Osteoporosis Risk Going Forward

Bone loss affects both density and structure, leading to weaker bones and an increased risk of fracture. As you get older, that can spell big trouble. In fact, every year in the United States 1.5 million people experience a fracture due to osteoporosis. The most common sites are the spine, wrist, or hip, but with osteoporosis, you can break a bone anywhere in your body even from a minor fall. Osteoporosis is responsible for more than 2.6 million doctor's office visits each year in the United States, and it can even result in hospitalization or having to live in a nursing home. Ninety percent of your bone mass is created by the time you're seventeen, but it's never too late to protect your bones and decrease your chances of getting a fracture. First, determine your risk factors.

Osteoporosis mostly affects women, but men might be surprised to learn that they are at risk too. Men generally have larger and stronger bones than women, but the National Osteoporosis Foundation estimates that two million American men have osteoporosis, and as many as twelve million are at risk for this disease. And although women lose bone mass more rapidly when they reach menopause, after age sixty-five, men and women actually lose bone mass at the same rate. The risk factors for men are similar to those for women, but low levels of testosterone can also increase men's odds for osteoporosis.

Risk factors for osteoporosis in both men and women include low calcium and vitamin D intake, not enough physical activity (especially weight-bearing exercise), smoking, heavy alcohol use, age, having a parent who had osteoporosis or broke a bone as an adult, being small and thin, and race (whites and Asians are at highest risk). Some chronic diseases, such as celiac disease, diabetes, and diseases affecting the kidneys, lungs, stomach, and intestines, or those that alter hormone levels, increase the risk for osteoporosis as well. Prolonged exposure to certain medications, such as steroids for asthma or arthritis, antiseizure drugs, some cancer treatments, some antidepressants, and aluminum-containing antacids, can also weaken bones.

Doctors use a bone mineral density (BMD) test to diagnose low bone density (osteopenia) or full-fledged osteoporosis. The National Osteoporosis Foundation recommends a central DXA (dual energy x-ray absorptiometry) test, which measures bone density in the hip and spine and takes less than fifteen minutes. Experts encourage all women over the age of sixty-five to have a BMD test, as well as younger, postmenopausal women who have risk factors, postmenopausal women who have stopped taking estrogen or hormone therapy, women going through menopause with certain risk factors, women who break a bone after fifty, and women with the diseases or who take any of the medications listed above. For men, your doctor might recommend a BMD test if you are between fifty and seventy and have one or more risk factors, are seventy or older even without any risk factors, have broken a bone after age fifty, or noticed a loss in height, sudden back pain, or a change in posture. Once you have a baseline BMD, your doctor can determine how often you need follow-up tests to measure changes in your bone density.

Preserve Your Bones for Years to Come

Armed with this information, you can control many of your risk factors. Besides quitting smoking (and avoiding secondhand smoke) and drinking only

moderately—if at all—make sure you consume enough calcium and vitamin D from food and supplements (▶ **42**, **43**), get plenty of exercise (▶ **38**, **39**, **40**), and maintain a healthy weight (▶ **41**). You can also make your home safer to protect against falls. For example, remove small rugs and items on the floor that you might trip over. Use nonslip mats in the bathtub and shower, and add handrails and good lighting in staircases. Wearing shoes with nonslip soles can also keep you more sure-footed. Ask your doctor whether your medications (even over-the-counter) or health conditions affect your bones and what other strategies you should enlist to protect your bones as you get older.

The Takeaway: Steps toward Better Bone Health

If you have risk factors such as advanced age, smoking, drinking alcohol, being small and thin, or having a history of osteoporosis in your family, request a bone mineral density test. Ask your doctor if any of your health conditions or medications could lead to bone loss.

Get enough calcium and vitamin D from foods and supplements.

Exercise regularly and maintain a healthy weight.

38

Step Up Your Strength Training to Reverse Age-Related Bone Loss

You already know that lifting weights is one of the best ways to stay trim, increase muscle mass, and rev up a slowing metabolism as you get older (▶ 20, 21). By preserving strength and muscle function, resistance training can also reduce your risk of falls and help you stay active doing the things you love. A wealth of research shows that it's also essential for staving off bone loss and keeping your frame strong well into later life. Bones are living tissues that continually grow and break down, but as you get older, you lose bone faster than you can regrow it (up to 1 percent per year after age thirty-five). Strength training helps fight bone loss because as weight pulls on your bones, it stimulates them to build new tissue and get stronger.

Lift Weights to Keep Bone Loss at Bay

Studies indicate that older adults who do strength training exercises can prevent bone loss and even build small amounts of bone, which can reduce the risk of potentially debilitating fractures. Most of the research has focused on postmenopausal women because they experience such a rapid loss of bone around the time of menopause, but a handful of studies show bone benefits for men as well. For example, a 2009 study in the *Journal of Strength and Conditioning Research* found that men who regularly did resistance training or high-impact aerobic exercise such as running had significantly higher bone mineral density (BMD) than those who were cyclists.

For women, however, menopause does pose a big bone risk, since your body no longer produces as much bone-building estrogen. In fact, during the five to seven years after menopause, women can lose up to 20 percent of their bone density, according to the National Osteoporosis Foundation. And while taking hormone replacement therapy (HRT) can help protect bones during this period of rapid loss, because of continuing concern over the health risks, many women are opting out of HRT. But menopause doesn't doom you to bone loss—a 2009 study by Brazilian researchers in the *Journal of Aging and Health* found that three strength training sessions a week preserved bone mineral density in postmenopausal women who were not taking HRT.

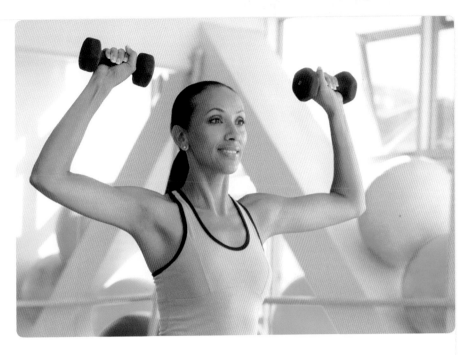

Adding to those findings, a 2009 study in the journal *Gynecological Endocrinology* followed a group of postmenopausal women with osteopenia (low bone density) or osteoporosis for one year and found that the women who did weight-bearing exercise slightly increased their bone mineral density (by 1.17 percent), while the control group who did not exercise lost 2.26 percent of their bone density. That's significant, because for every 1 percent of bone you rebuild, you reduce your risk of fracture by 5 percent.

Make Strength Training a Lifelong Habit

While researchers haven't determined the ideal exercise program to preserve and build bone, studies do give us some guidelines. For example, a 2007 review of studies in the *Journal of Geriatric Physical Therapy* determined that strength training helps maintain BMD in postmenopausal women and can increase the BMD of the spine and hip in women with osteopenia and osteoporosis. The review found the most benefit for "high loading" in weight training—working at 70 to 90 percent of maximum effort for eight to twelve repetitions per set, with two or three sets of exercises per session—and noted that people have to make exercise a permanent habit to continue seeing benefits and counteract "the chronic nature of bone loss." Other research shows that combining strength training with high-impact activities like running or climbing stairs (▶ **39**) is the best strategy for building bone.

For both women and men, it's wise to start building your bone bank as early as possible. For women especially, having normal bone density going into menopause will significantly reduce your risk of developing osteoporosis later in life. And you don't have to pump iron to strengthen your muscles. Lifting weights and using weight machines may be the most familiar methods, but you can also employ elastic exercise bands or use your own body weight for resistance, such as with yoga or Pilates, or in exercises such as push-ups, squats, and crunches. If you have osteopenia or osteoporosis, check with your doctor to determine the safest and most beneficial exercises for you.

The Takeaway: Resistance Training

You'll need to do three weight-bearing exercise sessions per week to build bone mass.

Work at between 70 and 90 percent maximum effort in two or three sets of eight to twelve repetitions each.

Use free weights, weight machines, or your own weight to perform resistance exercises.

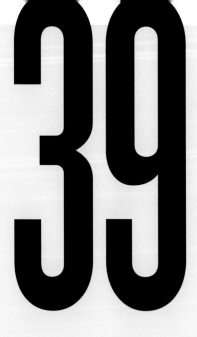

Add Weight-Bearing Aerobic Exercise to Keep Bones and Joints Young

Strength training is not the only way to build bones. Aerobic exercise that forces you to work against gravity and places weight on your bones and joints—called impact—may be just as important to preserve bone mass and prevent the decline in bone mineral density that you experience with age. University of Michigan researchers noted that exercise increases bone diameter by counteracting the thinning of bones and making them less porous. The pressure that these activities put on your bones sends a signal to your body to produce more bone cells and make your bones stronger, thus reducing the risk of fractures. As a bonus, strengthening your muscles helps you stay stable and can reduce stress on your joints. Regular exercise also nourishes cartilage and increases your range of motion, which is especially beneficial for people with joint pain.

Build Bones with High-Impact Activity As You Age

Although nonimpact activities like swimming and cycling do provide cardiovascular benefits, unfortunately, they don't seem to build bone. In fact, in a 2008 study in the journal *Metabolism*, male cyclists were seven times more likely to have osteopenia of the spine than runners, and they had significantly lower bone mineral density (BMD) of the whole body. To strengthen your bones, you need to put pressure on them. (A caveat: If you already have osteoporosis, high-impact activities may not be safe; ask your doctor for exercise suggestions.) Weight-bearing exercise can include walking, jogging, or running; using an elliptical trainer; racquet sports; stair-climbing; jumping rope; basketball; dancing; hiking; and soccer, among others.

A 2009 study in the *British Journal of Sports Medicine* suggests that a variety of impact exercises is most effective for preserving BMD, and combining weight-bearing aerobic activity with strength training provides the best benefits of all (▶ **38**). Intensity matters too. Walking, for instance, is generally considered low impact, but taking longer strides and walking at a faster pace provides more bone-strengthening force. Whatever activity you choose, when you strike the ground with your feet, keep your knees slightly bent to cushion your landing and protect your joints.

Of course, these kinds of activities also count toward your goal of thirty minutes of aerobic exercise on most (or all) days of the week to help boost a slowing metabolism (▶ **20**), keep your brain young (▶ **27**), lower your risk of heart disease (▶ **50**), and strengthen your immune system (▶66). You can still get bone benefits by breaking up your exercise into ten- or fifteen-minute blocks a few times a day. Or squeeze in bursts of bone-building activity throughout the day, like taking the stairs instead of the elevator to improve hip and leg bone strength (and burn a few extra calories while you're at it).

Exercise to Relieve Joint Pain

Whether you have a temporary ailment like tendonitis or bursitis (inflammation and swelling around the soft tissues of your joints), or a chronic condition like osteoarthritis (a breakdown of cartilage in the joint itself), experts agree that exercise can help. Aerobic exercise stimulates blood flow to joints, nourishing them and helping them stay flexible and elastic. A number of studies show that aerobic exercise (as well as strength training) helps manage osteoarthritis in mid- and late-life adults. Notably, a 2008 review of studies found that exercise improves physical function in people with knee osteoarthritis (OA) and reduces pain even as much as nonsteroidal anti-inflammatory drugs (NSAIDs) such as ibuprofen. Since these drugs have potentially serious side effects (▶48), exercise is a much better option to manage OA. Exercise can also help you stay at a healthy weight, reducing joint strain (▶41). And building muscle may actually reduce your risk of developing OA by relieving some of the burden on your joints as well.

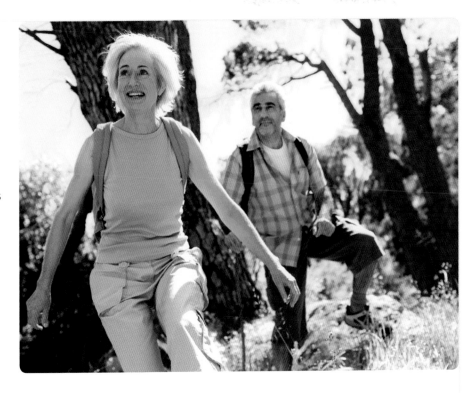

If you have painful joints, low-impact choices like walking might be easier on them, while still providing muscle-building and bone-strengthening benefits. You might feel a little stiffness as you move, especially as you begin, but stop if you feel pain. There is little evidence showing what types of exercise are most beneficial for osteoarthritis, but research suggests that solitary sessions, exercise classes, and home programs all provide similar gains. Your doctor can recommend activities that are safe for your sore joints.

The Takeaway: Aerobic Exercise for Your Bones and Joints

Activities that involve impact, like running and hiking, are better for building bone mass than nonimpact exercise like swimming or bicycling.

Combine high-impact aerobic exercise with weight training for maximum bone building.

If your joints are sore, exercise! It will flood them with nourishing blood.

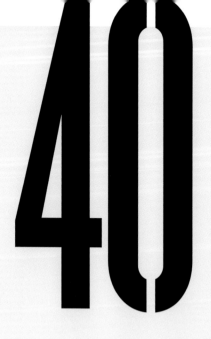

Improve Your Flexibility and Stability to Stay Limber

As you age, your risk of falling increases—and falls become potentially more dangerous because weaker bones raise your risk of getting a fracture (▶37). Besides being painful, those fractures are more likely to be in your spine or hip, which take a lot of time to heal and frequently result in hospitalization. In fact, one in five people with a hip fracture ends up in a nursing home within a year, according to the U.S. Surgeon General. But most falls are preventable, and since exercise simultaneously boosts muscle mass and strength, balance, and bone strength, it is one of the most important things you can do to protect yourself from falling as you get older.

Stretch to Stay Steady on Your Feet

Regular stretching increases your range of motion, improves balance, stabilizes muscles and joints, and helps prevent muscle injury. A 2009 study in the journal *Manual Therapy* found that even a single session of stretching exercises improved the stability and mobility of the female volunteers, allowing them to walk faster with longer steps—two variables linked to reduced risk of falling. A 2009 study in *Gerontology* looked at a similar stretching program performed for four weeks and found that by the end of the study, the older women had improved their hip and pelvis range of motion and could walk as well as healthy young adults. Stretching your abdominal and chest muscles can also perk up your posture, since stiff joints and tight muscles can literally pull you forward and give you a stooped appearance associated with being elderly.

Strive to stretch all your major muscle groups: calves, quadriceps and hamstrings, hip flexors, chest, and upper back. You may also want to stretch your neck and shoulders (especially if you sit for long periods), wrists, and ankles. Always warm up your muscles before stretching them, since stretching cold muscles can pull them and lead to injury. Move gently and slowly into a stretch until you feel gentle resistance, and don't bounce or hold your breath. Hold each stretch for thirty seconds. If you have osteopenia or osteoporosis, you should avoid stretches that involve flexing the spine or bending at the waist, since they may put too much stress on your spine and increase your risk of a compression fracture. Ask your doctor what stretches are best for you, or if you can modify certain stretches to make them safer.

Boost Your Balance to Reduce Risk of Falling

A 2003 study in the journal *Age and Ageing* followed a group of people over the age of sixty-five who were classified as being at risk of falling to see if exercise classes designed to help improve balance and muscle strength could help reduce the risk of falls. The participants attended an average of twenty-three classes over the course of a year and also did the exercises at home at least weekly. At the end of the year, the researchers found that those who took the classes scored significantly better on balance tests and had a 40 percent lower rate of falls than the control group who did not exercise.

Many kinds of exercise can help you balance better (▸ 23). Any weight-bearing activity that challenges the postural system can improve balance and potentially help reduce falls, according to the U.S. Department of Health and Human Services. But the most helpful might be dancing, yoga, Pilates, and tai chi, which improve balance, coordination, flexibility, and strength at the same time. Another advantage is that you can adapt the movements to fit your comfort level, and you can do them in your own home or in a group setting to get the benefit of social interaction. Community centers, adult education facilities, and gyms often offer organized programs and classes.

You should notice an improvement in balance and strength after about three months if you meet the goal of exercising (doing aerobic, strength, and flexibility activities) on most days of the week for at least thirty minutes. But remember that you have to keep at it to maintain those benefits!

The Takeaway: Better Balance

Dancing, yoga, Pilates, and tai chi are especially good exercises for balance, coordination, and strength.

You can do any of these at home, but taking a class combines the exercise with social interaction for a double benefit.

Keep working on your balance to maintain the benefits for life.

41

Maintain a Healthy Weight to Reduce Joint Stress and Protect Your Bones

Besides giving you an enviably youthful figure, staying within the normal weight range for your height is one of the best things you can do to protect your body against all kinds of age-related health problems, including cognitive decline (▶25) and heart disease (▶53). Your weight also affects your body mechanically (pressure on joints, effort required to move your limbs, etc.) and chemically (levels of circulating hormones, neurotransmitters, and other substances). So getting to—and staying at—a healthy weight is key to keeping all of your body systems in balance. And research shows it can also benefit your bones and joints.

Increase Muscle Mass to Keep Bones Strong

Being underweight increases your risk of osteoporosis and fracture. A 2010 study in the *Archives of Gerontology and Geriatrics* found that postmenopausal women who had a lower body mass index (BMI) and sarcopenia (age-related muscle loss) had correspondingly lower bone mineral content and density, possibly raising their risk of fracture. If you need to gain weight, you'll get the best bone and joint benefits by adding pounds of muscle rather than fat (▶38). Increasing muscle strength and control stimulates bone growth and helps stabilize your bones and joints to protect you from falls.

Start by calculating your resting metabolic rate (▶12). To gain one pound, you'll need to add an extra 3,500 calories to your diet. If you step up your strength training to boost muscle, you may need to eat more, since muscle burns more calories than fat. It may be tempting to turn to high-fat/high-carb foods like cake and croissants to increase calorie intake, but that approach will ultimately backfire by harming other aspects of your health (▶13, 25, 55). Instead, fill your plate with healthful higher-calorie foods that provide valuable nutrients, such as avocados, nuts, and olive oil. Protein-rich foods will also help you build and maintain muscle.

A regular regimen of strength training exercises that uses weights, elastic bands, or your own body weight for resistance is the best way to add muscle and ensure that the extra calories you take in don't convert to fat. Studies show that a strength training program can help you gain up to three pounds of muscle in just three months (▶21). Ask your doctor which strength training moves will help you safely and effectively put on muscle while protecting your bones and joints.

Lose Weight to Lighten the Load on Aging Joints

Being overweight increases the stress on your joints—each extra pound of weight you carry puts another three to four pounds of pressure on your knees and hips (because of the extra force exerted when your foot hits the ground), worsening pain, stiffness, and range of movement. Research shows that people with higher BMIs also tend to change their gait, walking more slowly and exerting greater impact forces because of the changes to their stride. But losing even a few pounds can relieve some of the burden on those hardworking hinges. A 2005 study in *Osteoarthritis and Cartilage* found that overweight and obese adults with knee osteoarthritis who lost 10 percent of their body weight increased their knee function by almost 30 percent.

In addition, excess body fat increases inflammation throughout the body, including in your joints. Inflammation not only makes joints more tender, stiff, and sore, but it may actually cause osteoarthritis to progress faster. Inflammatory substances circulating in your body can also affect muscle function and sensitize nerves, leading to increased pain. Researchers at the Wake Forest University School of Medicine found that obese adults over the age of sixty with knee osteoarthritis who lost as little as 5 percent of their body weight noticeably decreased inflammation throughout their bodies.

Adopting an anti-inflammatory eating pattern such as the Mediterranean diet can help you slim down (▶13) while also calming inflammation and tenderness in sore joints. However, losing weight can also cause bone mineral loss, weakening your bones and increasing your risk of fracture. Studies show that increasing your calcium intake while you're dropping pounds can help offset the loss of bone mineral, and adding a little more protein to the mix may further increase bone benefits, according to a 2008 study in the *Journal of Nutrition*. Plus, protein helps you hold on to metabolism-boosting muscle during weight loss (▶21).

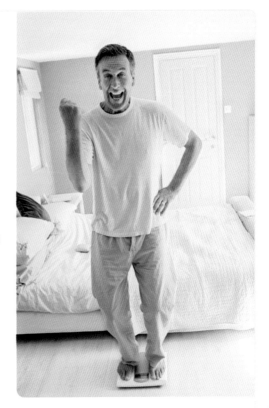

The Takeaway: Reach (and Maintain) a Healthy Weight

If you need to gain weight to stave off osteoporosis, choose quality calories such as fruits and vegetables, nuts and seeds, and healthy fats—not cake.

Combine a weight-gain program with strength training to ensure the extra calories don't get stored as fat.

If you need to shed extra pounds by eating less, avoid losing bone mass by increasing your calcium and protein intake.

42

Eat Right to Sustain Your Midlife Frame

Calcium may be the most critical component of a bone-healthy diet, but vitamin D, potassium, magnesium, and other nutrients play indispensable roles as well. So while you may think downing dairy is the only way to boost your bones, surprisingly, fruits and vegetables may be just as important because they supply so many other necessary nutrients. Studies show that eating more fruits and vegetables as part of a healthy eating plan, as in the Mediterranean and Dietary Approaches to Stop Hypertension (DASH) diets, can benefit your bones. A 2003 study in the *Journal of Nutrition*, for example, found that following the DASH diet for thirty days significantly reduced markers of bone turnover, which translates to less bone loss and lowered fracture risk. Add these bone builders to your diet to protect your frame as you get older.

Consume Enough Calcium and Vitamin D to Keep Bones Strong

The USDA's 2005 Dietary Guidelines for Americans recommends that adults get three servings of dairy or calcium-rich foods every day. Fortified foods like cereal, orange juice, soy milk, and tofu are also good sources. Adults up to age fifty need 1,000 milligrams of calcium per day, while after fifty you should aim for 1,200 milligrams per day. If you have osteopenia, your doctor may recommend getting as much as 1,500 milligrams from food and supplements combined. It's best to get your nutrients from food, but supplements can help make up the difference. Look for products marked "calcium carbonate" or "calcium citrate"; studies are mixed over which is absorbed better, but your doctor can help you decide which to take. Take no more than 500 to 600 milligrams at one time, and if you use iron supplements, don't take them with calcium, since calcium blocks iron absorption.

Vitamin D optimizes calcium absorption. Your body can make it when you expose your skin to sunlight, but for dark-skinned people or those in colder climates or heavily polluted areas who can't get outside every day, it's more practical to get the recommended amount through diet and supplements. U.S. dietary recommendations are 400 IU per day for adults age fifty to seventy, and 600 IU per day for those over age seventy. Fortified milk is the most common source of dietary vitamin D, but since manufacturers don't use fortified milk to make many other dairy products (such as cheese, ice cream, and most yogurts), those foods are not good sources. Check the nutrition facts label to verify the vitamin D content.

Increase Your Intake of Other Nutrients for Younger Bones

Potassium helps your bones conserve calcium, possibly by preserving the body's acid/alkaline balance. A 2009 study in the journal *Osteoporosis International* found that postmenopausal women who consumed the most potassium-rich foods had about 5 percent higher bone mineral density than those who consumed the least. Fruits and vegetables provide plenty of potassium, which researchers believe may be one of the main factors behind produce's bone benefits.

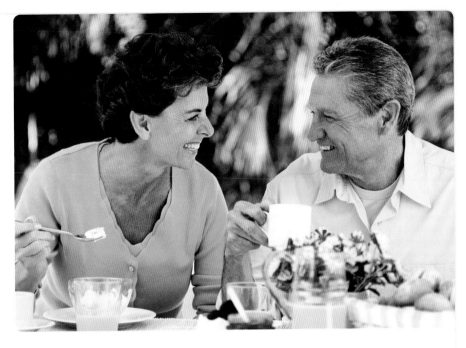

Magnesium increases calcium absorption and influences growth of crystals of hydroxyapatite, the mineral compound found in bone. Population studies have linked low magnesium intake to osteoporosis, and many people don't get enough. Find it in green leafy vegetables, whole grains, nuts, and dairy products.

"Vitamin C is essential for collagen formation and normal bone development," wrote Tufts University researchers in a 2008 study in the *Journal of Nutrition*. (Bones are one-third collagen, which gives them their flexibility.) They found that higher vitamin C intake protected against bone loss in older men, even if they had less-than-optimal calcium consumption. In a later study, the same researchers found that late-life men and women who consumed the most vitamin C (from food and supplements) significantly reduced their risk of fracture. Fruits and vegetables are your best sources for C and other antioxidants, including carotenoids such as beta-carotene and lycopene that protect against bone loss.

Research shows that vitamin K2 increases bone density and reduces fracture risk. Dark leafy greens, cruciferous vegetables, onions, and parsley contain vitamin K1, which your body can partly convert into beneficial K2 through digestion. Egg yolks, fermented dairy (such as cheese and yogurt), and fermented soy (such as miso and tempeh) are some of the few food sources of vitamin K2. Besides eating foods rich in K1 and K2, people with osteoporosis or osteopenia may want to supplement with 50 to 100 micrograms of K2 daily, and people with normal bone density may want to take 25 micrograms of K2. If you take anticoagulant drugs, check with your doctor before increasing vitamin K intake.

The Takeaway: Bone-Building Foods

Eat three servings per day of dairy or other calcium-rich foods, such as fortified cereal, orange juice, or tofu.

Eat plenty of fruits and vegetables to get potassium, magnesium, and vitamin C, which improve your body's ability to use calcium.

Egg yolks, cheese, and yogurt contain vitamin K2 (and your body can partly convert the K1 found in dark leafy greens, cruciferous vegetables, onions, and parsley), which can increase bone density.

43

Go Beyond Dairy for Bone-Building Calcium and Vitamin D

Although dairy products offer significant amounts of calcium and are frequently fortified with vitamin D, your bones may be better off if you get a good portion of these nutrients from nondairy sources. A 2009 review of studies in the *American Journal of Clinical Nutrition* noted that countries with the highest rates of dairy consumption also boast the highest rates of fracture from osteoporosis. That's not to say you need to shun cow's milk products entirely, since they are such a good source of calcium and, when fortified, vitamin D. But there's good evidence that filling your plate with a wide range of nondairy sources gives you the best bone benefit (good news for people who are lactose intolerant or who avoid dairy for other reasons).

Sup on Surprising Sources of Calcium to Keep Your Bones Strong

A 2005 study in the journal *Sports Medicine* found that after menopause, exercise's ability to boost bone mineral density (▶ **38**, **39**) largely depends on adequate availability of dietary calcium. Adults up to age fifty need 1,000 milligrams of calcium per day, and those older than fifty should aim for 1,200 milligrams per day. Vegetables, fish, and fortified foods offer nondairy alternatives to help you reach the recommended amounts.

Many vegetables contain calcium, but some have other compounds (such as oxalic acid) that inhibit calcium absorption. So while a half cup of cooked spinach serves up 115 milligrams of calcium, you'd need to eat sixteen servings to equal the amount of absorbable calcium you'd get in an 8-ounce glass of milk. Vegetables in the kale family (such as broccoli, bok choy, cabbage, and mustard and turnip greens) offer calcium that is as well absorbed as that in dairy products. One cup of cooked broccoli provides nearly 70 milligrams. Other good nondairy sources of calcium include dried figs, white beans, almonds, and edamame (fresh soybeans). Studies are mixed, but soy seems to increase bone density and prevent fractures after menopause, when the most dramatic bone loss occurs.

Canned sardines and salmon, with their tiny edible bones, also supply calcium. In fact, a 3-ounce serving of sardines contains more calcium (324 milligrams) than an 8-ounce glass of nonfat milk (302 milligrams)! Fortified orange juice, soy foods, and breakfast cereals also contain good amounts, and some may offer bone-building vitamin D as well.

Dine on Vitamin D–Rich Foods to Delay Bone Breakdown

Vitamin D is critical for calcium absorption (and science is beginning to discover its importance in other body systems as well). If you don't get enough, your body secretes too much parathyroid hormone, which speeds up bone breakdown. In fact, some studies show that increasing calcium intake alone is not sufficient to protect you from fractures as you get older: Vitamin D makes the difference. However, recent evidence indicates that a surprising number of people are deficient. Although your body can make vitamin D3 (cholecalciferol) from the UVB rays in direct sunlight, it's an unreliable source, and even some people who live in sun-soaked climates still don't make enough (not to mention rising concern about skin cancer risk). Plus, as you get older, your body is less efficient at producing vitamin D from the sun.

Few foods contain vitamin D, but salmon, mackerel, tuna, sardines, egg yolks, and fortified cereals are good sources. U.S. dietary recommendations are 400 IU of vitamin D per day in adults age fifty to seventy, and 600 IU per day in those over age seventy. In a 2008 study, Swiss researchers even suggested that all postmenopausal women and everyone over the age of sixty get 800 IU of vitamin D because it plays such a crucial role for bones and other aspects of health; other experts recommend that people who get very little sun exposure take as much as 1,000 IU per day. (Vitamin D is safe up to 2,000 IU, according to the Institute of Medicine.) To get that much, you'll almost certainly need to supplement in addition to eating these foods. Your multivitamin might contain some, and many calcium supplements now come with vitamin D as well. Look for D3 (cholecalciferol) on labels, since your body absorbs it better.

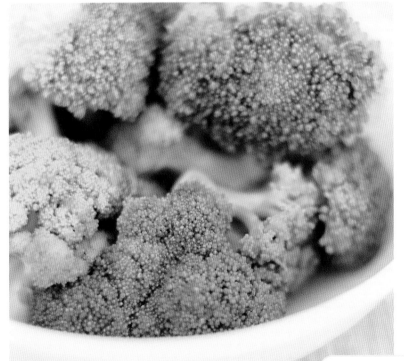

The Takeaway: Calcium and Vitamin D

Some vegetables, such as spinach, contain calcium but also other nutrients that inhibit absorption of calcium. Other vegetables, such as kale, broccoli, bok choy, and cabbage, are calcium powerhouses.

Vitamin D is necessary for calcium absorption. Foods such as salmon, mackerel, tuna, sardines, egg yolks, and fortified cereals are excellent sources.

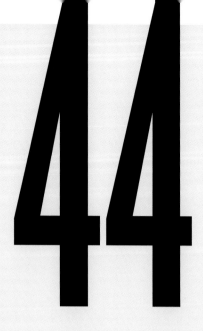

44

Heed These Diet Don'ts for Healthy Bones and Joints for Life

To protect your frame for the long haul, you need to do more than just eat foods rich in calcium, vitamin D, potassium, and other bone-benefiting nutrients. You should also minimize your intake of a few foods that can actually harm bone and joint health by triggering inflammation or leaching calcium from bones and blocking its absorption.

Pare Down Processed Foods to Protect Your Frame

Processed foods contain a variety of health-sapping substances, including trans fats, refined carbs and sugar, and sodium. While these things aren't necessarily good for you at any age, you'd do especially well to avoid them as you get older because of their harmful effects on your bones and joints.

Trans fats, processed carbohydrates, and sugar all increase inflammation in your body (▶ 25, 34), worsening stiffness, pain, and range of motion, and destroying cartilage in your joints. Inflammation also appears to accelerate bone breakdown and age-related bone loss. Sugar, in particular, has been implicated in increased osteoporosis risk, since it negatively affects the balance of minerals such as calcium and phosphorus needed for healthy bones. In animal studies, sugar has also been shown to decrease bone strength, potentially raising the risk of fracture. In general, experts recommend that you limit the amount of added sugars in your daily diet to less than 6 teaspoons (about 100 calories or 25 g) for women and no more than 9 teaspoons (about 150 calories or 37.5 g) for men (naturally occurring sugars, such as those in fruit and dairy products, are fine). You should also aim to eliminate trans fats entirely and swap processed carbs for whole grains whenever possible.

Excess sodium causes you to excrete more calcium, decreasing the amount available to bones. Sodium can also cause fluid retention and swelling, increasing pressure on tender joints. Manufacturers use salt and other high-sodium substances to preserve food and enhance flavor and texture, and processed and prepared foods such as canned vegetables, soups, deli meat, and frozen foods account for a whopping 77 percent of the average American's daily sodium intake. The USDA recommends limiting your sodium intake to 2,300 milligrams (one teaspoon of table salt) per day. By far, the easiest way to cut back is to reduce the amount of processed and prepared foods you consume.

Watch What You Drink to Age Well

Although research is mixed about whether caffeine increases osteoporosis risk, studies do show that caffeine can cause bone loss and may leach calcium from bones and interfere with calcium absorption. That's especially problematic for older adults, who need all the calcium they can get to preserve their bones. A 2001 study in the *American Journal of Clinical Nutrition* found that women over the age of sixty-five with high caffeine intakes had significantly higher rates of bone loss of the spine than did those with low intakes. A moderate intake (less than 300 milligrams per day) appears to be fine, but when you do consume caffeine, eat calcium-rich foods at other times to ensure maximum absorption of the mineral.

Sweetened beverages are bad for bones and joints because of their sugar content, which can lower bone mass and strength and aggravate inflammation. A 2008 study in the *Journal of Critical Care* found that soda drinkers, in particular, had reduced blood calcium and increased calcium excretion, setting them up for osteoporosis. Sugary soda that also contains caffeine is double trouble. But don't think you can simply reach for diet caffeine-free soda instead—a 2006 study in the *American Journal of Clinical Nutrition* found that even drinking diet and caffeine-free sodas a few times a week led to lower bone density in older women. Soda also contains phosphoric acid, which interferes with calcium absorption and contributes to imbalances that lead to additional loss of calcium. And nutrition experts point out that people usually drink sugar-sweetened or diet beverages in place of healthier sips such as water, milk, and tea, causing them to miss out on those beneficial drinks.

In addition to its other health benefits (▶ **26**), moderate alcohol intake appears to boost bone density. However, heavy drinking disrupts calcium balance in the bones, reducing bone mineral density and increasing risk of fracture. Alcohol can also aggravate some forms of arthritis, such as gout. Limit your intake to two drinks or less per day for men (one or less per day for women) for the best bone and joint protection.

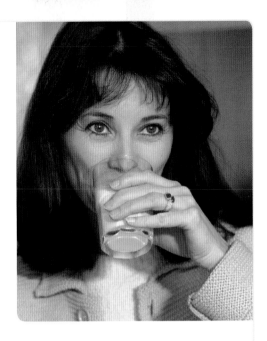

The Takeaway: Bone Destroyers

Sugar decreases bone strength and may contribute to osteoporosis. Consume a maximum of 6 to 9 teaspoons of added sugars a day.

Salt causes you to excrete calcium, leaving less available for bones. Avoid processed foods and limit your salt intake to one teaspoon (2,300 milligrams sodium) per day.

Caffeine leaches calcium from bones and interferes with its absorption. A little is okay (300 milligrams or less per day), but if you consume a lot of it, eat plenty of calcium-rich foods at other times to offset the risks.

Regular sodas contain sugar, caffeine, and phosphoric acid that destroy bone health (and diet options aren't much better). Drink water, milk, or tea instead.

45

Preserve Cartilage with Glucosamine and Chondroitin

Glucosamine and chondroitin sulfate are natural substances found in cartilage, the cushion between your joints. They first came to attention as potential osteoarthritis treatments when researchers speculated that supplementing with them would help rebuild cartilage worn down from wear and tear over the years. Glucosamine provides the raw material the body needs to manufacture long chains of sugar molecules (called glycosaminoglycans) found in cartilage and joint fluid. Chondroitin is the most plentiful type of glycosaminoglycan; it protects cartilage and attracts fluid to the connective tissue, bringing nutrients with it and allowing joints to absorb shock effectively.

As over-the-counter supplements, glucosamine and chondroitin are touted to help relieve symptoms of osteoarthritis (they don't seem to help other forms of joint pain and stiffness, such as bursitis or rheumatoid arthritis). In the last few years, several large studies have looked at the supplements in combination or separately, but they've found mixed results for effectiveness in easing pain and slowing the progression of osteoarthritis (OA). Part of the problem may be that researchers have used different forms of glucosamine in studies—both glucosamine sulfate and glucosamine hydrochloride are available. For example, preliminary evidence from a large study sponsored by the National Institutes of Health indicates that the combination of glucosamine hydrochloride (500 milligrams three times daily) and chondroitin sulfate (400 milligrams three times daily) helps treat moderate to severe knee OA pain, but doesn't relieve milder pain. This combination also failed to forestall the joint degeneration of OA.

However, a 2002 study in the *Archives of Internal Medicine* followed a group of people with knee OA and found that those who took 1,500 milligrams of glucosamine sulfate every day for three years slowed the progression of the disease and improved pain, function, and stiffness. And a 2007 review of studies in the journal *Drugs and Aging* suggests that chondroitin sulfate combined with glucosamine sulfate—as opposed to glucosamine hydrochloride—is more likely to help improve OA symptoms. They also found "compelling evidence" that glucosamine sulfate and chondroitin sulfate stabilize cartilage loss and slow joint degeneration. So if you'd like to try these supplements, the evidence points to glucosamine sulfate and chondroitin sulfate as being your best bet.

Supplement to Ease Age-Related Joint Pain

Most people with osteoarthritis can safely take 1,500 milligrams of glucosamine and 1,200 milligrams of chondroitin daily, the amount used in studies. Bump up the dose to 2,000 milligrams glucosamine and 1,600 milligrams chondroitin if you weigh more than 200 pounds (90.7 kg). You may want to divide the doses and take them throughout the day with food to prevent nausea and increase absorption. Allow three months to notice an improvement (some experts even suggest giving them six months).

These supplements are safer than other pain-relieving drugs like NSAIDs (aspirin, ibuprofen, and naproxen), which can cause ulcers and stomach bleeding if taken long-term, and COX-2 inhibitors such as Celebrex, which have been linked to cardiovascular problems (▶48). Another plus: Research indicates glucosamine and chondroitin may even be more effective than Celebrex. Still, talk to your doctor before taking glucosamine and chondroitin, since they may interact with drugs like diuretics and blood thinners. You should avoid chondroitin supplements made from shark cartilage, since they could be contaminated with heavy metals. And if you have a shellfish allergy, read ingredients labels carefully, since most glucosamine supplements are made from shellfish covering.

Since glucosamine and chondroitin are considered supplements, they are not regulated like drugs in the United States. That means that there is no guarantee that claims made on the label are accurate, or that the supplement contains the amount of active ingredient it claims to (if any). Select supplements from well-known manufacturers to increase the likelihood that they contain the stated amount and are free from contamination. You can also check the subscription-only Consumer Lab website (www.consumerlab.com), which offers independent testing of popular supplements by a variety of manufacturers.

The Takeaway: Glucosamine and Chondroitin

Studies vary with regard to the efficacy of this popular combination, but evidence suggests that glucosamine sulfate and chondroitin sulfate can relieve pain and stiffness and may even slow the progression of OA.

Split the doses and take the supplements with food to avoid nausea and boost absorption.

Glucosamine and chondroitin may interact with diuretics and blood thinners.

Avoid chondroitin supplements made from shark cartilage, since they may contain heavy metals; most glucosamine supplements are made from shellfish coverings, so read the label if you have a shellfish allergy.

46

Try Natural Remedies to Strengthen Older Joints

Glucosamine and chondroitin may get all the press (▶45), but there are other natural remedies that can help alleviate joint stiffness and pain. And because they carry less risk of harmful side effects than traditional treatments like nonsteroidal anti-inflammatory drugs (NSAIDs) and COX-2 inhibitors (▶48), these supplements might just deserve a spot in your medicine cabinet.

Supplement with SAM-e to Soothe Sore Joints

Short for S-adenosylmethionine, SAM-e occurs naturally in cells. Your body produces less of it as you get older, which caused researchers to wonder if supplementing could help conditions like osteoarthritis (OA) and other joint pain. Scientists suspect that SAM-e relieves pain by calming inflammation, and it may help keep cell walls flexible and allow for better cell communication as well. SAM-e also spurs production of the antioxidant glutathione, quelling free radicals. Lab and animal studies have shown SAM-e can stimulate the production of cartilage, but more research is needed to see if it can do the same in humans.

Studies show SAM-e can reduce joint pain and stiffness seemingly as well as traditional pain relievers like NSAIDs and COX-2 inhibitors. For example, researchers at the University of California, Irvine, compared SAM-e (1,200 milligrams) with celecoxib (Celebrex 200 milligrams) for sixteen weeks to see how they reduced pain associated with knee OA. The researchers found that after two months, both treatments improved pain and joint function equally, although SAM-e took longer to take effect.

It's expensive to take the full recommended dose of SAM-e, although many people find that after an initial period of high dosing they can maintain the effects with a smaller amount. Start with 400 milligrams three times a day for two weeks, then decrease to 200 milligrams twice a day thereafter. People taking SAM-e seem to tolerate it well and are less likely to report problems than people using NSAIDs, but SAM-e can have side effects at the high dose, such as mild digestive distress (though it doesn't damage your stomach, like NSAIDs can do). Choose enteric-coated products labeled "butanedisulfonate," which is the most stable form. Some research suggests SAM-e also has an antidepressant effect, so unless your doctor says it's okay, you shouldn't use it if you are taking antidepressant medications to avoid interactions.

Try Pycnogenol to Relieve Arthritis Pain

Researchers believe pycnogenol, the patented name for a French maritime pine bark extract, helps OA by fighting free radicals (it contains potent antioxidant compounds called bioflavonoids) and calming inflammation. A 2008 study in the journal *Phytotherapy Research* found that OA sufferers who took 100 milligrams of pycnogenol daily for three months had significantly reduced pain and stiffness and better joint function, and could walk much farther on a treadmill test compared to those given a placebo. What's more, pycnogenol takers were able to cut back on other pain-relieving medications such as NSAIDs and COX-2 inhibitors by 58 percent (and had 63 percent fewer gastrointestinal side effects as a result!). In a similar study published later that year, patients with mild to moderate OA took 150 milligrams of pycnogenol daily and also experienced pain relief significant enough to allow them to reduce NSAID use.

Pycnogenol seems to be safe and well tolerated, but talk to your doctor if you'd like to try it, since it also has cardiovascular effects and could reduce your need for hypertension drugs. It may affect your blood sugar levels as well. Take 50 milligrams two or three times daily with meals.

Herbal Help for Healthy Joints

A handful of small studies indicate that extracts of *Boswellia serrata* (frankincense), an anti-inflammatory herb, help calm inflammation and improve OA symptoms such as pain, swelling, and joint function. A 2007 study in the *Indian Journal of Pharmacology*, for example, compared boswellia extract (1,000 milligrams daily, divided into three doses) with a COX-2 inhibitor and found that, while boswellia didn't take effect as quickly, within two months both treatments had similar benefits on OA symptoms. And the people who took boswellia continued to notice improvements for up to a month after stopping the treatment, whereas the COX-2 inhibitor's effects dwindled as soon as that group stopped taking the drug. A recent lab study also showed boswellia prevented cartilage degradation. But more and better-designed studies in humans are needed to gauge the herb's benefit. As a 2008 review of studies in the *British Medical Journal* noted, "The evidence for the effectiveness of *Boswellia serrata* extracts is encouraging but not compelling."

The Takeaway: Natural Painkillers

SAM-e, while expensive, reduces OA joint pain as well as the need for NSAIDs, which may have harmful side effects.

Pycnogenol, a pine bark extract, fights free radicals and calms inflammation, reducing pain and stiffness.

Boswellia serrata, an anti-inflammatory herb, may relieve pain and swelling even up to a month after you stop taking it.

47 Reduce Midlife Joint Pain with Alternative Therapies

Beyond exercising (▶39, 40), staying at a healthy weight (▶41), eating well (▶44), and taking supplements (▶45, 46), some complementary approaches have shown promise for improving joint pain and other osteoarthritis symptoms. Acupuncture, transcutaneous electrical nerve stimulation, and massage can be helpful add-ons to other treatments and may be effective enough to allow you to reduce or even eliminate pain medications. Ask your doctor if it's worth giving these therapies a shot; insurance may cover or subsidize them.

Consider Acupuncture to Reduce Age-Related Stiffness

Acupuncture is probably the best-studied alternative therapy for treating joint pain and osteoarthritis (OA). Originating in China, acupuncture developed as a technique for restoring the balance of energy, or qi, in the body.

Practitioners insert thin needles in points of the body that correspond to painful areas; the resulting stimulation of nerves, muscles, and connective tissue releases your body's natural painkillers (called endorphins), suppresses stress hormones such as cortisol, and boosts blood flow. Electro-acupuncture is a common variation that uses pairs of needles and mild, continuous electric pulses traveling between them to provide additional stimulation.

Studies on acupuncture show a small, short-term benefit for pain, but because of the difficulty of devising a placebo treatment, the actual effect has proved tricky to measure. Still, the results are promising. A 2008 review of studies in the journal *Family and Community Health* concluded that acupuncture is effective for improving pain and joint function in knee OA. And a 2010 study

in the *Chinese Medical Journal* found that people with knee OA who received electro-acupuncture had reduced pain and several improved measures of joint function, including step length and walking pace.

Acupuncture has very few side effects and is considered quite safe if your practitioner is certified and uses sterile needles in a clean environment. However, you'll have to continue treatment to keep seeing results.

Try Out TENS to Block Pain Signals

Similar to electro-acupuncture, transcutaneous electrical nerve stimulation (TENS) uses a small, battery-powered machine with electrodes you attach to your skin to send a low-voltage electrical current along nerve fibers. These electrical impulses stimulate the nerve

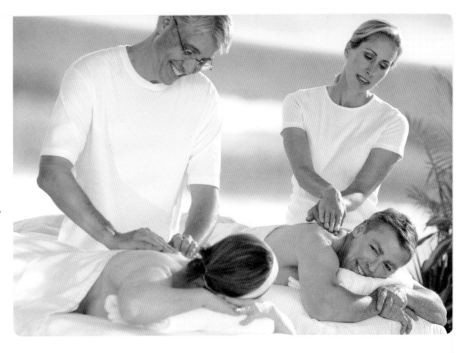

endings near painful joints, potentially blocking pain signals to the brain and triggering a release of endorphins. After initial training on how to use the machine, you can do the therapy at home. It's generally considered safe.

Several small trials have indicated that TENS can help relieve pain due to knee OA. And based on a review of current research, the Osteoarthritis Research International group, a team of sixteen medical professionals from six different countries, includes TENS as one of its twelve recommended nondrug treatments (along with acupuncture) to manage hip and knee OA.

A 2008 study in the *American Journal of Physical Medicine and Rehabilitation* found that combining hot packs and TENS reduced pain and improved function in women with knee OA. The TENS treatment group also showed increased muscle strength and better exercise performance compared to those who received ultrasound therapy plus hot packs, hot packs alone, or no treatment. And in a 2008 study in the journal *Chinese Medicine*, knee OA sufferers reported less pain and improved joint function after treatment with TENS. Those researchers found similar improvement with acupuncture and suggested that combining TENS and acupuncture would provide even greater benefits.

Massage for Greater Range of Motion and Joint Strength

Massage is helpful in reducing pain and increasing joint range of motion and strength. It works by encouraging blood flow to joints and stimulating endorphin release, and it may diminish pain-worsening stress hormones like cortisol as well. Because there are at least eighty different kinds of massage, gathering conclusive evidence about its effects on joint pain has proved difficult. However, a 2006 study in the *Archives of Internal Medicine* found that Swedish massage (twice weekly for a month, then weekly for another month) significantly improved knee pain, stiffness, and joint function in OA sufferers compared to those who didn't receive massage. With very little downside, and potential benefits beyond relieving OA symptoms (it feels so good!), health-care practitioners frequently recommend massage to alleviate OA pain.

The Takeaway: Alternative Therapies for Joint Pain

Acupuncture relieves pain by releasing endorphins, suppressing stress hormones, and boosting blood flow—without harmful side effects.

TENS devices block pain signals and trigger the release of endorphins, your body's natural painkillers.

Massage improves pain, stiffness, and joint function, and it feels wonderful!

48

Discuss Arthritis and Osteoporosis Drug Side Effects with Your Doctor

Osteoarthritis pain not only interferes with your quality of life, but it can actually worsen joint function if left untreated. If you have pain, you're probably tempted to limit your movements, but that can backfire by tightening, shortening, and weakening the ligaments, tendons, and muscles that move your joints. That means less mobility and function over time, which is exactly what you don't want as you get older. Enter pain relievers.

Osteoporosis, on the other hand, is often called a silent disease because it generally has no symptoms, until you break a bone. It's natural to want to protect your bones, and bone-saving drugs promise to do that. But no medication is perfectly safe; being informed can help you find the right treatment and hopefully avoid distressing side effects.

The Dangers of Drugs for Osteoarthritis

When used as directed, acetaminophen can relieve joint pain from osteoarthritis (OA) with few side effects. But some people find (and most studies agree) that nonsteroidal anti-inflammatory drugs (NSAIDs) such as aspirin, ibuprofen, and naproxen work better. Just because they're over-the-counter, however, doesn't mean they're without risk. Evidence shows that long-term use of aspirin and ibuprofen can lead to gastrointestinal problems like ulcers and bleeding, and naproxen may lead to heart trouble. People with a history of gastrointestinal bleeding (such as stomach ulcers), kidney insufficiency, or heart failure, or who are taking blood thinners, should not use NSAIDs. If you do take them regularly, and long-term, your doctor may want to monitor your kidney function and also recommend

that you take an acid-reducing medication like omeprazole to protect against stomach ulcers.

Pain relievers called cyclooxygenase-2 (COX-2) inhibitors were developed to be safer for your stomach, and they appear to be as effective as nonprescription NSAIDs. But studies have linked COX-2 inhibitors to increased risk of heart problems and stroke, prompting the makers of Vioxx and Bextra to pull those drugs off the market in 2004 and 2005, respectively. Another popular COX-2 inhibitor, Celebrex, remains available but with a warning label about cardiovascular risks. If you decide to try either nonprescription NSAIDs or COX-2 inhibitors, follow the package instructions and take the lowest possible dose—and be patient, since it may take a few weeks before these drugs effectively manage your pain.

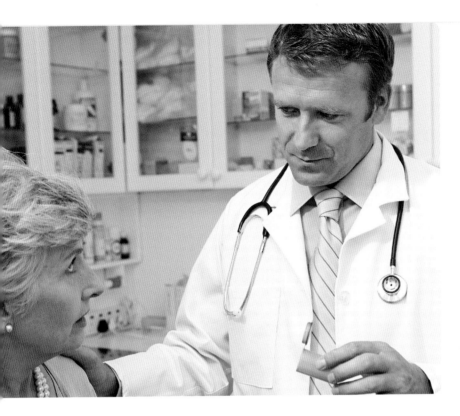

The Takeaway: Drug Dangers

NSAIDs work better than acetaminophen to relieve joint pain, but they may cause ulcers, gastrointestinal bleeding, and heart problems.

COX-2 inhibitors can lead to heart problems and stroke.

Bisphosphonates have potentially serious side effects, including severe joint pain, esophageal reflux, cancer, heart problems, destruction of the jawbone, and spontaneous fracture.

The Unintended Consequences of Osteoporosis Medicines

Popular osteoporosis drugs such as Fosamax and Boniva belong to a class of drugs called bisphosphonates, which can help boost bone mass and reduce fracture risk in people with low bone mineral density. People who have had an osteoporotic fracture, have taken corticosteroids, or are frail can benefit from bisphosphonates, but potentially serious side effects lead some experts to suggest that widespread use of these drugs is not the best approach to prevent or treat osteoporosis. Several recent studies warn about the risks of bisphosphonates, including severe bone, joint, and muscle pain; esophageal reflux; and even cancer. The U.S. Food and Drug Administration is also investigating a connection to irregular heartbeat. Ironically, the drugs have also been linked to destruction of the bone in the jaw and spontaneous fracture, often in the femur (the long thigh bone), possibly because the drugs appear to strengthen the outer cortical bone but not the trabecular bone, the inner lace-like structure that gives bones their incredible tensile strength.

Although most of these side effects are rare, bisphosphonates accumulate in bone and are released for months or years after treatment is stopped, so it's worth discussing these potential risks—and their early warning signs—with your doctor if you're thinking about taking them. In a 2010 study in the *Journal of Clinical Endocrinology and Metabolism*, researchers suggested that people who take the drugs long-term schedule a "drug holiday" for a few years, even recommending that people with low risk of fracture only take bisphosphonates for five years and then stop entirely as long as bone mineral density stays stable and no fractures occur. In the meantime, bone-saving strategies like exercise (▶ **38, 39**) and eating well (▶ **42, 43, 44**) are safe and effective and may reduce your need for osteoporosis drugs as you get older—and it's never too late to start these healthy habits!

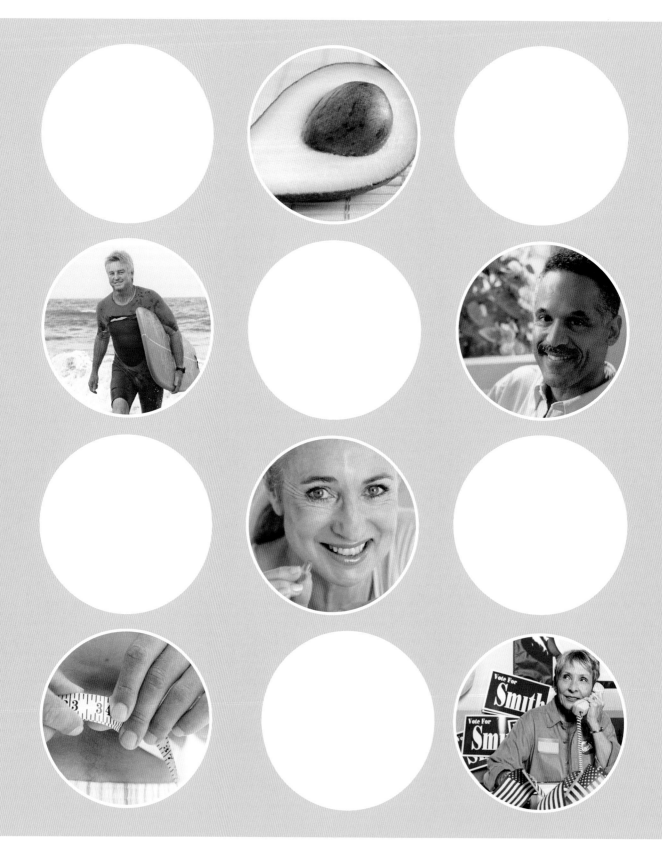

PART V

Turn Back the Clock on Your Heart

49

Request New Tests to Determine Age-Related Risk Factors

Heart disease is the number-one worldwide killer of men and women, and your risk of cardiovascular problems increases as you get older. Doctors look at a constellation of health markers to help determine your likelihood of having a heart attack over the next ten years. Called the Framingham Risk Score, this tool was developed using data from thousands of people over several decades, and the results are fairly reliable. Beyond these traditional indicators, scientists have discovered new ways to pinpoint the presence of heart and vascular disease and have recently developed tests that can provide additional information about your risk.

Find Your Framingham Score for Risk of Heart Attack

Besides age, other unchangeable factors like gender and race play a role in your risk. Black men, for example, appear to have the highest chance of dying from cardiovascular disease. And women's risk increases significantly after menopause. But there are several critical elements that you can control, including your cholesterol levels (▶51), blood pressure (▶52), diabetes (▶55), and tobacco use (▶93).

Cholesterol levels tend to increase as you get older, and the higher your total, the higher your risk for heart disease. According to the American Heart Association, adults should aim for less than 200 mg/dL total cholesterol. In addition, your doctor will test other blood lipids, such as triglycerides, to get a better picture of your overall risk. Doctors recommend keeping your systolic blood pressure (the top number) below 120 mm Hg and your diastolic blood pressure (the bottom number) below 80 mm Hg for the best cardiovascular health. Although diabetes is defined as having fasting blood glucose of 126 mg/dL or more, some evidence indicates that prediabetes, or fasting blood glucose between 100 to 126 mg/dL, also ages your heart. And of course you'll want to reduce (and ideally eliminate) all exposure to tobacco smoke. To get a picture of your overall cardiovascular risk, the Cleveland Clinic offers an easy-to-use Framingham Risk Score calculator at http://my.clevelandclinic.org/ccforms/Heart_Center_Risk_Tool.aspx.

Take Other Tests for Various Heart Risk Markers

In addition to the Framingham Risk Score, a few new tests measure substances called cardiac biomarkers in your blood, which can give a clearer indication of your odds for developing cardiovascular disease. That information can help you and your doctor decide how aggressively to treat the risk factors you have, helping to ensure that your heart stays young and healthy. Talk to your doctor about whether you're a good candidate.

A high-sensitivity C-reactive protein (CRP) test measures the concentration of a plasma protein that increases with inflammation. Since inflammation likely contributes to buildup of plaque in your arteries (atherosclerosis), a CRP test may provide an early warning for people already at risk for cardiovascular disease. Anything above 3.0 mg/L indicates high risk.

Homocysteine is an amino acid naturally found in the blood, and high levels are linked to coronary artery disease, stroke, and peripheral vascular disease. Homocysteine is normally higher in men than in women and increases with age. Your doctor may order the test if you have a family history of heart disease, or if you've had cardiovascular problems but don't have traditional risk factors, such as smoking. Normal levels are 0.54 to 2.3 mg/L.

Lipoprotein(a) is a type of LDL cholesterol based more on genetics than lifestyle, and experts believe it can contribute to atherosclerosis and heart disease. If you have atherosclerosis but normal cholesterol levels, a family history of early-onset heart disease or sudden death, or if cholesterol-lowering drugs aren't working for you, request a lipoprotein(a) test in addition to regular LDL screening. The risk of elevated lipoprotein(a) depends on your LDL cholesterol level, but a result of 80 mg/dL or higher warrants treatment.

High levels of fibrinogen, a protein that helps your blood to clot, make it more likely for clots to form in an artery, reducing blood flow to the heart and raising your risk of stroke. It's also a marker of inflammation, which can speed up atherosclerosis. However, the test can't identify the source of the inflammation, so doctors only perform it when you're already at risk for heart disease. Normal levels are between 200 and 400 mg/L.

Another test is called cardiac calcium scoring, which uses a CT scan to measure the buildup of calcium in plaque in the arteries of your heart. Normally you shouldn't have any; if you do, it's a sign of coronary artery disease. Most doctors don't recommend this test unless you have a 10 to 20 percent chance of having a heart attack in the next ten years (considered medium risk) based on your other risk factors.

The Takeaway: Heart Tests

Calculate your Framingham Risk Score to determine your chance of having a heart attack in the next ten years.

Request other tests to measure heart biomarkers, including CRP, homocysteine, lipoprotein(a), fibrinogen, and cardiac calcium scoring.

50

Exercise Regularly to Keep Your Heart Young

Your heart is a muscle, and like other muscles in your body, it gets weaker as you age unless you exercise to strengthen it. Exercise directly affects your likelihood of developing heart disease and, at the same time, improves other risk factors such as cholesterol (▶51), blood pressure (▶52), weight (▶53), and diabetes (▶55). Work up to doing thirty to sixty minutes of exercise (aerobic and strength) on most days of the week. Can't squeeze that much into a single session? Research shows you'll still reap heart benefits by breaking up your activity into ten-minute bursts throughout the day. By making physical activity a lifelong habit, you can stave off future heart problems and keep your heart young, healthy, and functioning its best for years to come.

Get Your Heart Pumping for Younger Blood Vessels

There's a reason aerobic exercise is often referred to as "cardio." Aerobic exercise dilates your blood vessels and keeps them flexible, combating age-related stiffening, improving blood flow, and making it easier for your heart to pump blood throughout your body. Any kind of activity that raises your heart rate is good—dancing, rowing, skating, tennis, basketball, jogging, skiing, and cycling, to name a few—but walking is perhaps the most popular. Walking is easy and inexpensive, and you can adjust your speed to your fitness level. A 2002 study published in the *New England Journal of Medicine* found that brisk walking for just two and a half hours a week cuts your risk of heart attack and stroke by nearly a third. And in this case, more is better—exercising five hours a week slashes your risk in half!

Exercise can also help you recover from heart trouble and reduce the risk of further problems. A 2004 study in the journal *Circulation* followed a group of one hundred men diagnosed with heart disease. Researchers directed some of them to do twenty minutes of cycling per day, and the others received an angioplasty (surgery to clear a blocked artery and prop it open with a tube called a stent). The exercise group had a 90 percent chance of being free of heart problems one year later, compared to only 70 percent of those who got the procedure. What's more, the exercise group had fewer trips to the hospital and cut their treatment costs in half.

Convinced you should lace up your sneakers? Pick up the pace for better heart health; to get the cardiovascular benefits of exercise, you want to reach 65 to 85 percent of your maximum heart rate. To find that range, subtract your age from 220. Next, multiply the answer first by 0.65 and then by 0.85 to get the bottom and top numbers you should aim for. Track your pulse using a heart rate monitor or by stopping to check periodically (press your fingers against the artery on the side of your neck under your jaw and count the number of beats for six seconds, then multiply that number by ten). A simpler way is to perform the "talk test." If your breathing is somewhat hard while you're exercising but you can talk without gasping for air, you're in the target zone. Always end your workout with a cooldown, gradually slowing your pace until your heart rate falls below 65 percent of your maximum, to prevent a dangerous drop in blood pressure.

Pump Iron to Boost Blood Flow

Strength training also keeps blood vessels young and flexible while increasing blood flow. It can help your heart work more efficiently and reduce cardiovascular risk factors as well. A 2009 study found that patients with mild heart failure who did strength training three times a week for eight weeks improved several markers of heart function compared to those who received standard care. And researchers at the University of Maryland found that regular strength training reduces your resting blood pressure over time.

Since resistance training can spike your blood pressure while you're performing

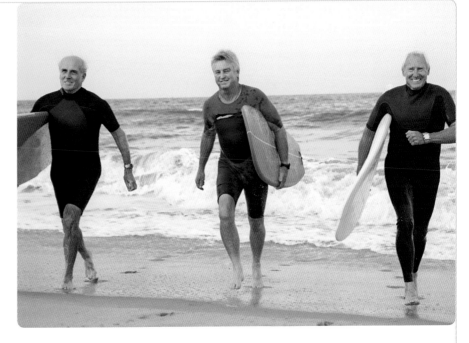

the exercises, if you have hypertension or are at risk for heart problems, check with your doctor before starting a strength program. Some research indicates that training at a low intensity (40 to 60 percent of your maximum capability) with more repetitions only modestly raises blood pressure while working out. For most people, with or without cardiovascular disease, the benefits of strength training far outweigh the risks.

The Takeaway: Heart-Healthy Exercise

Work up to doing thirty to sixty minutes of aerobic exercise per day to reduce your risk of heart disease, high cholesterol, high blood pressure, excess weight, and diabetes.

Walking for five hours a week reduces your risk of a heart attack by 50 percent.

Lift weights three times a week at about half your maximum capacity to prevent a spike in blood pressure.

51

Lower Your Cholesterol Naturally

Your risk of cardiovascular disease increases as you get older, partly because cholesterol levels rise with age until you reach age sixty or sixty-five. Experts recommend keeping your total below 200 mg/dL; high levels (240 mg/dL and above) double your risk of heart disease. But total cholesterol doesn't tell the whole story. There are actually thirteen different kinds of cholesterol, including four types of low-density lipoproteins (LDL—the "bad" cholesterol), and they each play a different role in cardiovascular health. A full lipid panel test reveals more about your risk of heart disease and the best way to keep cholesterol levels in check.

For high-density lipoproteins (HDL), the "good" kind that keeps cholesterol from building up in the walls of the arteries, the higher the numbers, the better. Less than 40 mg/dL is considered a major risk factor for heart disease, while 60 mg/dL and above actually protects against heart problems. Women often have higher HDL than men.

LDL accumulates in your arteries and creates fatty deposits called plaques that reduce blood flow. Rupturing of those plaques can cause serious heart and vascular problems. Ideally, your LDL should be less than 100 mg/dL (levels of 160 to 189 mg/dL are considered high), but women's LDL levels often rise with menopause.

Triglycerides are another type of blood fat that usually results from eating more calories than you burn (one reason why being overweight increases your risk of heart attack). High levels have been linked to coronary artery disease. You want your triglycerides to be less than 150 mg/dL.

If your cholesterol is high, you may not need to add another medicine to your regimen to get your levels back into a safe range. Talk to your doctor about trying these natural approaches (give them about three months to show results) before taking a cholesterol-lowering drug that carries side effects. And even if you're already taking a cholesterol medication, these strategies can improve its effectiveness, potentially allowing you to reduce your dose.

Adopt Lifestyle Changes to Live Longer

As you get older, your weight tends to creep up (▸12). Excess weight lowers HDL while raising LDL and triglycerides, but losing as little as 5 to 10 pounds (2.3 to 4.6 kg) can help reverse that effect. One of the most effective dietary changes you can make is to reduce your intake of refined carbohydrates such as white flour and sugar, and processed foods, which provide empty calories that get converted into triglycerides (and extra pounds). Eat more whole grains, legumes, fruits, and vegetables for their cholesterol-clearing fiber and plant stanols and sterols, which lower LDL. Swapping out saturated and trans fats for healthier monounsaturated fats—found in olive and canola oils, avocados, nuts, and seeds—and omega-3s (▶ **25, 58**) is another smart step.

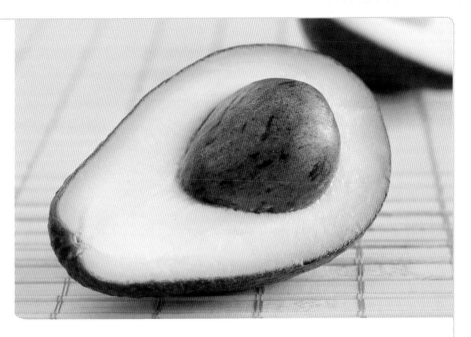

Whether or not you're overweight, regular exercise can boost HDL and lower triglycerides. In fact, exercise is one of the few things capable of boosting heart-protective HDL. And if you are carrying a few extra pounds, exercise can help you lose weight, thereby lowering LDL. A 2009 study in the *Journal of Physical Activity and Health* found that previously sedentary men who began exercising significantly improved measures of HDL, LDL, and triglycerides in just eight weeks. Aim for thirty to sixty minutes of moderate activity on most or all days of the week.

Supplement to Lower Cholesterol

Artichoke leaf extract (*Cynara scolymus*) may reduce total cholesterol with few mild and quickly disappearing side effects, according to a 2009 review of studies. Preliminary research suggests it might also reduce LDL and triglyceride levels, but more studies are needed to

confirm that effect. Take 1,800 to 1,920 milligrams a day, divided into two or three doses.

If you butter your bagel (whole grain, of course) every day, consider switching to a margarine that contains plant stanols and sterols, which can reduce total cholesterol and LDL. Look for beta-sitosterol or sitostanol, found in margarines like Promise Activ or Benecol.

Fiber supplements like blond psyllium (found in seed husk and products such as Metamucil) and oat bran also help lower total cholesterol and LDL, and ground flaxseed can help reduce triglycerides. For every 1 to 2 grams of soluble fiber you consume daily, you may lower your LDL by 1 percent, according to the Cleveland Clinic. Increase your fiber intake slowly to avoid digestive distress, but women should aim for 25 grams and men for at least 30 grams daily.

The Takeaway: Lower Cholesterol without Drugs

Reduce your intake of refined carbohydrates such as white flour and sugar, and processed foods.

Eat whole grains, legumes, fruits, and vegetables.

Exercise at a moderate pace for thirty to sixty minutes on most days of the week.

Switch to a margarine that includes plant stanols and sterols.

Supplement with artichoke extract and fiber.

52

Control Your Blood Pressure without Drugs

High blood pressure is one of the most common conditions among middle-aged and older adults, affecting more than 900 million adults worldwide by some estimates. Blood pressure is the force of blood against the walls of arteries, and it's recorded as two numbers: systolic (as the heart beats) and diastolic (as the heart relaxes between beats). For the best heart health, your blood pressure should be below 120 systolic and 80 diastolic, as measured in millimeters of mercury (mm Hg). A reading of 140/90 mm Hg or higher is considered high.

Also called hypertension, high blood pressure ages and hardens your blood vessels and makes your heart work too hard—it is a major risk factor for cardiovascular disease. In fact, for every 20 mm Hg systolic or 10 mm Hg diastolic increase in blood pressure, your chances of dying from cardiovascular disease

double. High blood pressure often has no signs or symptoms, so it's critical that your doctor checks your blood pressure at least every two years. If you have high blood pressure, or if you have a history of heart disease, get it checked more frequently. Simple lifestyle changes can help lower your blood pressure and prevent hypertension, or keep existing high blood pressure under control.

Eat a Heart-Healthy, Low-Sodium Diet to Lower Blood Pressure

A wealth of evidence shows that eating plans that emphasize fruits, vegetables, and low-fat dairy and are also low in sodium, saturated and trans fat, total fat, and cholesterol can lower blood pressure. One such plan, called Dietary Approaches to Stop Hypertension (DASH), also highlights whole grains, poultry, fish, and nuts, and limits fats, red meats, sweets, and sugary drinks. Ease

into this style of eating by serving two or more meatless meals per week, snacking on fruits and vegetables, and serving fruit for dessert. Reducing the amount of meat and other high-fat ingredients in your favorite dishes is another painless way to improve your diet. In your famous lasagna, for example, switch to part-skim mozzarella, use half the ground beef, and add spinach, broccoli, and roasted red peppers to the filling.

Sodium is a big factor in blood pressure for many people. Eating a lot of salt holds excess fluid in your body and increases the burden on your heart, wearing it out faster. And while setting down the salt shaker can help, the vast majority of our sodium comes from prepared and processed foods such as canned vegetables, soups, deli meat, and frozen foods. The USDA recommends limiting your sodium intake to 2,300

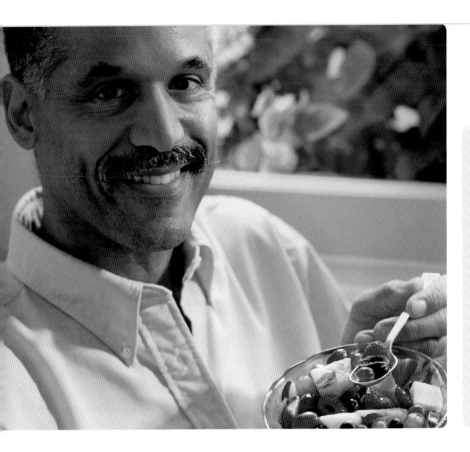

milligrams (1 teaspoon of table salt) per day, but if you have high blood pressure, your doctor may recommend cutting back even further. A 2001 study in the *New England Journal of Medicine* found that reducing sodium intake to 1,500 milligrams per day had the biggest blood pressure benefits. To cut down on sodium, eat fewer processed foods and be diligent about reading nutrition labels on the packaged foods you do eat, and try flavoring foods with herbs instead of salt.

Alcohol also increases blood pressure, and imbibing more than one drink per day for women, or two for men, may lead to hypertension. One drink is equal to 12 ounces (360 ml) of beer, 4 ounces (120 ml) of wine, 1.5 ounces (45 ml) of 80-proof distilled spirits, or 1 ounce (30 ml) of 100-proof spirits.

Get Moving to Prevent and Control Hypertension

Researchers have known for a long time that exercise is key to preventing hypertension. But until recently, the evidence was less clear that physical activity could improve existing high blood pressure. Now new research, including a 2010 study in the *Journal of Sports Sciences*, has confirmed that regular aerobic exercise and strength training reduce blood pressure across the board. In a 2006 review of studies, the researchers found that people with high blood pressure got the biggest benefit from exercise, reducing their systolic number by almost 7 points and their diastolic by nearly 5 points. People with normal blood pressure also lowered their measurements, by 1.9 points systolic and 1.6 diastolic, decreasing the likelihood that they would develop high blood pressure as they got older. As a bonus, exercise can also help you lose weight, reducing another risk factor for hypertension.

53

Watch Your Waistline to Protect Your Heart for Life

It probably comes as no great shock that being overweight increases your chances of developing heart disease. Being overweight places extra stress on many of your body's systems, aging you and worsening several risk factors for heart disease, including cholesterol (▶51) and blood pressure (▶52). But what might surprise you is just how much your weight is a factor: A startling one-third of all fatal cardiovascular diseases can be attributed to excess weight and obesity, and about one in seven nonfatal cases, estimated Dutch researchers in a 2009 study in the *European Journal of Cardiovascular Prevention and Rehabilitation*.

One way doctors gauge your risk of heart disease is by measuring your body mass index (BMI). You can find a BMI calculator online, or you can measure it yourself by dividing your weight in kilograms by the square of your height in meters (kg/m²). Overweight is defined as having a BMI between 25 and 30, while a BMI greater than or equal to 30 translates to obesity (or being about 30 pounds [14 kg] overweight for a 5'4" woman). How much weight you've gained over the years also matters: Results from the Nurses' Health Study show that those who gained between 22 and 42 pounds (10 and 19 kg) since they were eighteen were 2.6 times more likely to develop cardiovascular disease, while those who gained 44 pounds (20 kg) or more upped their odds 7.4 times.

Some evidence shows that an even more important number than your BMI or the reading on the scale is your waist measurement. Carrying your weight around your middle—where excess pounds usually settle as you get older (▶12)—significantly increases your risk of heart disease and diabetes (which itself is a major risk factor for cardiovascular problems). If your waistline measures more than 40 inches (102 cm) for men and more than 35 inches (88 cm) for women, which fits the definition of obese, you need to take action. A pair of recent studies by German and U.K. researchers found that another indicator of abdominal fat, having a waist-to-height ratio of greater than 0.5, is also better at estimating your risk of heart disease than BMI. (The researchers estimated that 17 percent of all men and 6 percent of all women are in the normal BMI range but still carry their weight around their middle, which actually puts them at higher risk of cardiovascular disease than being overweight but having those extra pounds spread out more evenly). Their advice: "Keep your waist circumference to less than half your height."

Start Shedding Pounds for a Longer Life

If you are too heavy or have fallen prey to middle-age spread and need to shrink your waistline, you'll be encouraged to know that even small improvements have big payoffs for your heart. For example, losing as little as 5 to 10 pounds (2.3 to 4.6 kg) can help raise your HDL (the "good" cholesterol) while lowering LDL and triglycerides. And dropping 10 pounds (4.6 kg) reduces your blood pressure.

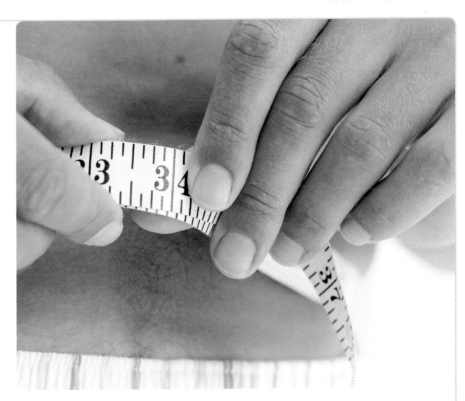

So how do you get started? First, figure out how many calories you really need to eat per day (▶12). Once you know your daily calorie needs, following an anti-inflammatory eating pattern, such as the Mediterranean diet (▶13), not only helps you drop pounds but can calm heart-damaging, aging inflammation as well. With the emphasis on fruits and vegetables, whole grains, beans, fish, and healthy fats, you won't have as much room in your diet for calorie- and fat-laden, nutritionally empty foods that not only pack on pounds but increase your risk of diabetes.

Next, bump up your physical activity. Aerobic exercise helps torch calories (▶20), strength training increases metabolism-boosting muscle (▶21),

and sneaking more movement into your everyday life can burn hundreds of extra calories virtually effortlessly (▶22). But remember, to lose weight and keep it off, you have to both watch what you eat and move more. As important as exercise is to your heart and to rev up a sluggish midlife metabolism, it's a lot easier to avoid eating an extra 200 calories of bread at dinner than it is to burn it off later!

The Takeaway: Waist Watchers

Know your measurements: Calculate your BMI and waist-to-height ratio to gauge your risk of heart disease.

Lose weight if you need to; dropping even 5 or 10 pounds makes a huge difference in the stress on your heart.

It's as simple as it sounds: Exercise more and eat less.

54

Get the Nutrients You Need to Stave Off Heart Disease

Some of the healthiest foods for your heart are fruits and vegetables, nuts, and whole grains, according to a 2009 study in the *Archives of Internal Medicine*. These superstars offer key nutrients like antioxidants, B vitamins, and fiber, which help fight age-accelerating free radicals, improve heart and blood vessel function, and clear out artery-clogging cholesterol.

Amp Up Your Antioxidant Intake for a Stronger Heart

Plant foods are rich in free radical–fighting antioxidants called flavonoids, and diets that emphasize them are linked to lower death rates from cardiovascular disease, likely because the antioxidants improve the function of the endothelium, the smooth inner lining of the heart and blood vessels. Your endothelium stops working as well as you get older, and oxidative stress from free radicals speeds up that decline.

Preliminary lab studies suggest that free radicals may also be responsible for dislodging plaques that have formed in blood vessels, potentially leading to a blockage and subsequent heart attack or stroke. And a 2009 study in the *Journal of Clinical Biochemistry and Nutrition* found that people with existing cardiovascular disease might be even more susceptible to the damaging effects of free radicals.

For heart health, vitamins C and E, carotenoids (such as beta-carotene and lycopene), and resveratrol are a few standout antioxidants. Vitamin E (found in wheat germ, nuts and seeds, and vegetable oils) prevents free radicals from attacking blood fats, and vitamin C (in citrus fruits, kiwi, and red and green peppers) relaxes blood vessels to boost blood flow while regenerating vitamin E. Low levels of carotenoids (sources

include carrots, cantaloupes, sweet potatoes, and spinach) are linked to atherosclerosis, a buildup of plaque in blood vessels. And resveratrol, found in grapes and wine, acts directly as an antioxidant to relieve oxidative stress on the endothelium, but a 2009 study in the *Journal of Physiology and Pharmacology* found that it also boosts the performance of other important antioxidants in the body. Evidence is mixed for supplements, but research clearly shows a heart benefit to boosting your intake of antioxidant-rich plant foods: Eat five to nine servings a day.

Bring on the B Vitamins to Reduce Stress and Inflammation

A 2010 study in the *American Journal of Clinical Nutrition* found that low vitamin B6 concentrations are connected to inflammation, increased oxidative stress, and metabolic conditions such as obesity and diabetes. Studies link low blood levels of folic acid with a higher risk of dying from heart disease and stroke. And B vitamins—particularly folic acid, B6, and B12—reduce levels of homocysteine, an amino acid linked to cardiovascular problems (▶ **49**). Homocysteine increases with age, and it seems to accelerate atherosclerosis by damaging the inner lining of arteries and promoting blood clots. Surprisingly, studies that have looked at supplementing with B vitamins to lower homocysteine levels show inconsistent results about their benefit to heart health. But experts agree on the importance of getting enough B vitamins in your diet to prevent heart problems and keep blood vessels young and healthy.

The American Heart Association recommends getting 400 micrograms of folic acid a day. Citrus fruits, tomatoes, green leafy vegetables, and grain products are good sources, as are some fortified foods. You can find B6 in fortified cereals, beans, meat, poultry, fish, and some fruits and vegetables (over the age of fifty, men need 1.7 milligrams daily, and women need 1.5 milligrams). Adults need 2.4 micrograms of vitamin B12 per day, but as you get older you may not be able to absorb it as well; ask your doctor if this is a concern for you. Animal products, including fish, meat, poultry, eggs, and milk, are good sources of B12.

Feast on Fiber for Lifelong Benefits

The two types of dietary fiber, soluble and insoluble, each have benefits for your heart. Soluble fiber can lower LDL ("bad") cholesterol, modestly lower blood pressure, and reduce heart disease risk. Insoluble fiber not only reduces the likelihood that you'll develop heart disease, but also it can actually slow the progression of heart problems in high-risk people. Eating high-fiber foods also makes you feel fuller, helping you keep your weight in check. Women should aim for 25 grams a day and men for at least 30 grams, but build up to that amount gradually to avoid stomach problems. Whole grains such as oats, barley, and brown rice are generally good sources of dietary fiber, as are beans, peas, carrots, cauliflower, apples, and nuts.

The Takeaway: Nutrition for Heart Health

Eat five to nine servings a day of antioxidant-rich plant foods that are high in vitamins C and E, carotenoids, and resveratrol.

Citrus fruits, tomatoes, green leafy vegetables, and grain products are good sources of folic acid; fortified cereals, beans, meat, poultry, fish, and some fruits and vegetables contain vitamin B6. Animal products such as fish, meat, poultry, eggs, and milk provide B12.

Fill up on soluble and insoluble fiber from whole grains, fruits, vegetables, and legumes.

55

Dodge Diabetes As You Age by Decreasing Sneaky Sugars

After you eat, your blood glucose (blood sugar) rises and your pancreas produces insulin to help muscle, fat, and liver cells use that blood glucose for energy. If your body does not make enough insulin or cannot use it well—called insulin resistance—high levels of glucose build up in your blood, setting the stage for diabetes. Having a cluster of any three controllable risk factors—insulin resistance, being overweight (especially around your middle), high blood pressure, HDL ("good" cholesterol) levels below 35 mg/dL, and triglyceride levels above 250 mg/dL—is called metabolic syndrome, and it dramatically increases the likelihood that you'll develop diabetes.

Type 2 diabetes is perhaps the most aging condition there is. Besides putting you at high risk for heart attack and stroke, having high blood sugar damages nearly every system in the body over time. For example, the high levels of insulin produced in response to excess blood sugar also act on your kidneys (raising your blood pressure), influence the liver enzymes that produce cholesterol, and increase inflammation throughout your body.

Your doctor can use a fasting blood glucose test to check your blood sugar levels in the morning after eight hours of not eating. Normal blood sugar levels are 100 mg/dL or less. Prediabetes, classified as having blood sugar levels of 100 mg/dL to 125 mg/dL, is also dangerous to your heart, but you still have time to turn things around and prevent full-blown diabetes. Diabetes is defined as blood sugar levels of 126 mg/dL or higher.

Most people with prediabetes go on to develop type 2 diabetes within ten years, unless they lose 5 to 7 percent of their body weight (about 10 to 15 pounds [4.5 to 6.8 kg] for someone who weighs 200 pounds [90 kg]) through diet and exercise. Research shows that lifestyle changes are twice as effective at preventing diabetes as medications, and one of the most important changes you can make is to decrease your sugar intake to help keep your blood sugar, insulin levels, and weight in check.

The Dangers of Age-Accelerating Added Sugars

Not all sugar is bad. Some foods, like fruit and milk, contain natural sugars that your cells can use for energy. But they also contain fiber and protein, respectively, to help balance out your blood sugar and prevent an insulin spike. Added sugars are the real problem because they typically break down very quickly and increase your blood sugar too fast—and they're not always easy to sleuth out. You know to limit obvious offenders like soft drinks, cookies, cakes, ice cream, and doughnuts to once-in-a-while treats. Same with sprinkling brown sugar on your oatmeal or pouring syrup on your pancakes. But your morning cereal, canned or frozen fruit, canned baked beans, spaghetti sauce, and other seemingly healthy foods can be sneaky sources of added sugars, even if they don't taste especially sweet!

The only way to tell if a food has added sugars is to look at the ingredients list. And sugar by any other name tastes just as sweet: Look for names ending in "ose," such as maltose or sucrose, high fructose corn syrup, molasses, cane sugar, corn sweetener, raw sugar, syrup, honey, or fruit juice concentrates. The American Heart Association recommends limiting the amount of added sugars to no more than 100 calories per day, or about 6 teaspoons (24 g) of sugar, for women. For men, stick to 150 calories or less per day, or about 9 teaspoons (36 g). That's a drastic cut from the typical American intake of 22 teaspoons (88 g) of sugar a day—about 355 calories! Clearly, added sugars are adding to our waistlines as well.

Another problem with foods high in added sugars is that they're often nutritionally empty, so including them in your diet likely means you're missing out on beneficial foods that can improve your health and slow aging. In addition to reducing your added sugar intake, improve your overall dietary picture by eating more whole grains, beans, fruits, and vegetables. Besides being filled with fiber, which can lower your insulin levels, these foods also contain complex carbohydrates, which take longer to break down and cause a more gradual rise in blood sugar while still providing energy to cells.

The Takeaway: Stealthy Sugars

Limit soft drinks, ice cream, and baked goods to once-in-a-while treats; the same goes for syrup on your pancakes, honey in your tea, and other added sweeteners.

Read the label to find hidden sugars in packaged foods like cereal, canned fruit, canned beans, and spaghetti sauce.

Limit your daily intake of added sugars to 6 teaspoons (24 g) for women and 9 teaspoons (36) for men.

56

Tame Stress and Anger to Take Years off Your Ticker

You wear many hats throughout your lifetime, and trying to fill several roles at once—spouse, parent, caregiver, friend, employee/retiree—can be exhausting. In fact, over time the small daily stressors wear on us more than sudden, devastating events. Chronic stress ages your heart by increasing heart rate, blood pressure, and blood sugar and continually flooding your body with cortisol. High cortisol levels are linked to atherosclerosis, the buildup of plaque in the arteries, according to a 2008 study in the *Journal of Clinical Endocrinology and Metabolism*. In addition to the ways stress directly harms your heart, it can also tempt you to try other risky behaviors, such as smoking, drinking, overeating, or using drugs to relieve pressure.

Anger is a common response to stress, and evidence shows it can spike your heart rate and blood pressure, potentially raising your risk of heart problems. However, while early research showed that anger in general is harmful for your heart, new studies suggest that how you express your anger matters more. For example, a 2009 study in the *British Journal of Health Psychology* demonstrated that suppressing anger has immediate and delayed cardiovascular consequences. In addition, a 2010 study in the *American Heart Journal* found that men and women who blamed others for their anger increased their heart disease risk as much as 31 percent. Men in the study who discussed their anger to resolve a situation, on the other hand, lowered their chances of developing heart disease.

The studies on anger illustrate an important truth: Since our lives will likely always contain some chaos, our focus needs to be on responding well to stressful situations. And that pays dividends beyond keeping your heart healthy and young—it can also help you get more satisfaction out of your now-longer life! To deal with anger in a healthy way, choose your battles and resolve to fight fair (don't be nasty, sarcastic, domineering, or hit below the belt, and avoid body language such as rolling your eyes). Above all, don't suppress your anger and stew about it—that's a recipe for heart disaster. Find a trusted confidant you can vent to, but use the conversation to help you move past anger, not dwell on it.

Reduce Stress Where You Can to Live Longer, Happier

While you can't entirely eliminate stress, you can employ strategies to minimize certain triggers. For example, if long lines at the grocery store send your stress levels skyrocketing, try shopping at a less busy time. Or if a coworker or relative gets on your nerves, cut back on the time you spend around him or her. Another key is to be realistic about what you can and can't (or want to) fit into your schedule—then practice tactful ways of saying "no" to avoid overcommitting yourself. And when you have a mile-long to-do list, prioritize your tasks to ensure that you have enough time to tackle the most important things. Items that don't get done can shift to another day (or you may eventually realize that you can let them go!).

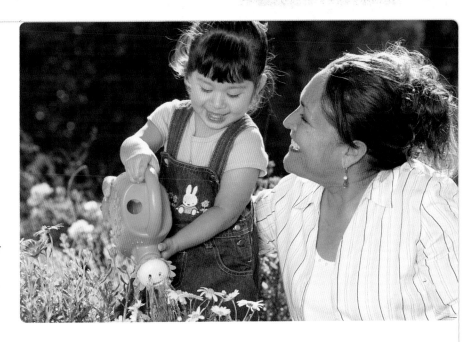

Change Your Response to Stress for Long-Lasting Benefits

Exercise changes your body's reaction to stress by keeping your stress hormones balanced and boosting your mood (▶4). That can make all kinds of pressure-filled situations easier to bear. Getting enough sleep can help you handle stress better as well. Also, give yourself time to decompress daily by doing things you enjoy, whether it's pursuing a hobby, listening to music, or playing games with friends or loved ones. Even setting aside five minutes in the morning and in the evening to take a few deep breaths can help.

Cultivating happiness, or an optimistic outlook, helps tame tension, and research shows it can benefit your heart as well. Consciously choosing to look for the positive in situations can help you reframe your thoughts and break out of a negative spiral, notes Jason F.

Mathers, Ph.D., a licensed psychologist in private practice. It can also help you identify aspects you have control over and can work to change, like asking your spouse to take over caring for an aging parent one day a week. Laughter is another powerful stress buster, and research shows it can buffer stress's effects on blood pressure and help the inner lining of your blood vessels stay flexible and function better.

The Takeaway: Stress Busters

If you're angry, discuss it; don't let it stew. Be direct without being mean.

Know your limits: Reduce the time you spend with people who push your buttons, and don't overschedule yourself.

Look on the bright side, get plenty of sleep, and pursue your hobbies to relieve stress.

57

Become a Volunteer and Live Longer

Volunteering offers a multitude of health benefits, including keeping your heart young and strong. Whether it's due to fostering friendships and combating depression or providing an enjoyable way to increase your physical activity, volunteering pays rich health dividends for you while helping your community at the same time. From museums to community centers, all kinds of organizations depend on volunteers, so you're sure to find one that matches your interests and skills (or helps you learn something you've always been interested in!). You can reap the health benefits by volunteering just two hours a week, or about 100 hours a year, according to the Corporation for National and Community Service. Find a service opportunity at www.VolunteerMatch.org, or if there's a specific place you'd like to volunteer, ask at the front desk how you can get involved.

Volunteering Keeps You Socially Engaged As You Age

"If I had to pull out the biggest benefits of volunteering, it would be social connection and fighting depression," says Sarah Lovegreen, M.P.H., health manager with OASIS, a national organization that promotes lifelong learning and service for adults age fifty and older. Depression increases your chances for heart problems even aside from traditional cardiovascular risk factors such as hypertension, high cholesterol, increased body mass index, a history of cardiovascular issues, and disease severity, notes a 2009 study in the journal *Stress*. And other evidence indicates that social isolation—common in older adults, and a key factor in depression—can double your risk of dying from coronary artery disease.

Just how depression affects your heart is less clear, although some research suggests it might increase inflammation, influence clotting, and affect your autonomic nervous system, which is responsible for raising or lowering your heart rate, constricting blood vessels, and increasing blood pressure. Scientists aren't yet sure whether treating depression reduces risk of cardiovascular disease and death, but early evidence shows that selective serotonin reuptake inhibitors (SSRIs) might help.

A 2009 study in the journal *Age and Ageing* found that older adults who volunteered or continued working past retirement age had fewer depressive symptoms, better mental well-being, and greater life satisfaction than those who retired without volunteering. And a 2010 study in the *Journal of Aging and Health* found that volunteering actually helps lift depression in people over sixty-five years old.

Volunteering helps combat depression by giving you a sense of purpose and connection, which is especially valuable if you don't currently get that from a job. Being socially active has a cyclical benefit too—if you connect with others, it can reduce depression, which in turn makes you more likely to stay socially engaged.

Volunteering Keeps You on Your Toes

Volunteering is a great way to boost your physical activity and stay young. A 2009 study in the *Journal of Urban Health* found that older adults who volunteered fifteen or more hours a week in an elementary school described themselves as having increased strength and energy and were able to walk and climb stairs faster than before they began volunteering. Another study looking at the same group of volunteers found that they burned almost twice the calories of their nonvolunteering counterparts, and they sustained that higher level of physical activity over time. That extra exercise, even if it's not enough to qualify as your daily workout, can benefit your heart (▶50).

If you're retired, or thinking about retiring, volunteering can help you stay active. A 2007 study in the *American Journal of Epidemiology* found that people who retired lost the work-related physical activity (such as transportation to and from work) formerly built into their day, and they didn't make up for that change by increasing participation in sports or other leisure-time activities. Other research shows that even when retirees continue with sports and exercise participation, they also increase the time they spend in sedentary activities like watching television. Volunteering gets you up off the couch, and the additional movement in your daily routine might be enough to offset an aging metabolism (▶22), helping you stay slim and reducing a key risk factor for heart disease.

The Takeaway: Volunteering

Volunteering helps your health as well as the community. Match your interests with the needs of a museum, school, or other organization.

Volunteering fights depression by keeping you socially engaged. It gives you a sense of purpose and identity, which you might not be getting from a job.

Volunteering keeps you physically active, helping you stay fit, fighting depression, and giving you more energy.

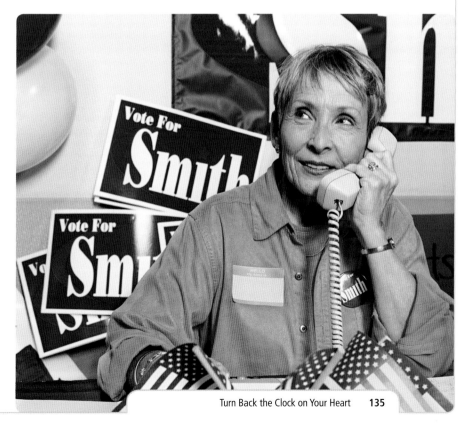

58

Use Supplements to Strengthen Your Cardiovascular System

In addition to taking supplements targeted directly at specific risk factors, such as high cholesterol (▸51), solid science suggests a few supplements are good for overall heart health. If you're at high risk for heart disease, or if you already have cardiovascular problems, ask your doctor if you could benefit from taking these supplements.

Omega-3s Offer Anti-Aging Benefits

The omega-3 fatty acids eicosapentaenoic acid (EPA) and docosahexaenoic acid (DHA) are found in oily fish such as salmon, mackerel, herring, lake trout, sardines, and albacore tuna, and study after study continues to extol their anti-aging effects (▸3, 25). While they show particular promise for people with prior heart disease or who are at high risk for cardiovascular problems, they also seem to benefit the hearts of healthy

people. A 2009 review of studies in the *American Journal of Therapeutics* noted that strong evidence shows omega-3s can lower triglyceride levels, slow plaque buildup in your arteries (atherosclerosis), modestly lower your blood pressure, and protect against abnormal heartbeats and heart attack.

If you don't get your omega-3s through food, you can supplement with fish oil capsules. Some research has raised concern about possible contamination with mercury, dioxins, and industrial chemicals called PCBs in fish oil supplements. Purifying reduces or removes these contaminants, and independent research by ConsumerLab .com and the Environmental Defense Fund notes that most well-known brands meet strict safety requirements. Some supplements state on their labels that PCBs and other contaminants have

been removed. You can also check the Environmental Defense Fund website, EDF.org, for a list of manufacturers' ratings in independent tests, or search for contaminant-free brands in the International Fish Oil Standards database (www.ifosprogram.com).

The American Heart Association recommends that most people get 500 milligrams of EPA and DHA per day for heart health (whether from fish or fish oil capsules). Discuss your dose with your doctor, but studies show that people with coronary artery disease should take 1 gram per day, and those with high triglycerides should take 2 to 4 grams per day, divided into three doses. If you're vegetarian, choose a supplement with DHA from algae, or take up to 3 grams of flax oil (your body can convert some of its alpha-linolenic acid to omega-3s). Fish oil breaks down when exposed to light and heat, so look for a brand with natural preservatives like vitamin E or rosemary, purchase supplements from a store with high turnover, and store them in the refrigerator or freezer. To reduce fishy aftertaste and burps, take the capsules at the beginning of a meal and swallow them frozen.

Consider Coenzyme Q10 to Keep Your Heart Young

Coenzyme Q10 (CoQ10) is a fat-soluble, vitamin-like substance found in every human cell. Responsible for producing energy, it also acts as an antioxidant and can benefit your brain (▶ **36**) as well as your heart. CoQ10 is naturally present in a variety of foods, including beef, soybean oil, sardines, mackerel, and peanuts, but people at risk for cardiovascular disease will likely need to supplement to get enough to see its heart-protective effects.

Studies show that CoQ10 benefits the heart by maintaining healthy blood vessels, preventing plaque buildup and reducing the risk of plaque rupture, supporting the heart cells' high energy requirements, and protecting LDL ("bad") cholesterol from a process called oxidation that makes it harmful to blood vessels. A 2009 review of studies suggested that CoQ10 might help lower blood pressure as well. Additionally, preliminary evidence indicates that it may help treat congestive heart failure when used alongside other conventional treatments, although more research is needed to determine CoQ10's role. Cholesterol-lowering statin drugs can suppress production of CoQ10, which may cause the fatigue and muscle and joint aches that some people experience while taking the medicines (▶ **59**). A 2007 study in the *American Journal of Cardiology* found that supplementing with 100 milligrams per day of CoQ10 reduced those side effects.

Anyone who is taking statins, who has a family history of heart problems, or who is otherwise at risk for cardiovascular disease may benefit from supplementing. Take 50 to 150 milligrams per day in softgel capsule form, and for best absorption, take it with a meal containing fat.

The Takeaway: Supplements for Your Heart

Eat oily fish (salmon, trout, mackerel, sardines, and tuna) to get the heart-healthy benefits of omega-3s. If you don't eat enough fish, supplement with fish oil capsules, preferably frozen and with a meal to reduce fishy aftertaste and burps.

Take CoQ10 to increase energy and fight heart-aging free radicals. CoQ10 also benefits the heart by reducing plaque buildup and the risk of plaque rupture.

59

Combat the Aging Side Effects of Heart Medicines

If you have risk factors for heart disease, such as high cholesterol, high blood pressure, or diabetes, your doctor has probably prescribed medicine to help control the condition. While these drugs are generally safe and well tolerated, they can have troublesome side effects—sometimes severe enough to make people stop taking the medications. In other cases, these drugs cause nutritional deficiencies that don't show symptoms right away, but can speed aging and lead to significant health problems over time. Talk to your doctor right away if you experience any of these side effects, and try the following strategies to reduce symptoms and replenish depleted nutrients.

Stop Statins' Heart-Aging Side Effects

These popular cholesterol-lowering drugs, such as Lipitor, can cause headache, digestive distress, and muscle and joint pain. They also block the body's production of the antioxidant coenzyme Q10 (CoQ10), which is important to many aspects of heart health (▶58), including fighting free radicals that accelerate cardiovascular aging, helping heart cells use oxygen efficiently, and keeping blood vessels young, flexible, and healthy. A deficiency of CoQ10 can cause fatigue, and it may be responsible for the aforementioned muscle and joint pain statin users sometimes experience. A 2009 study in the journal *Current Drug Safety* notes that rare statin side effects include liver dysfunction, reducing the ability of the heart muscle to contract properly, rapid muscle breakdown, and peripheral neuropathy, a disease marked by pain, tingling, numbness, and loss of sensation in the extremities.

Experts agree that the benefits of statins often outweigh the risk of side effects in people who are not able to lower their cholesterol through lifestyle changes (▶51). If you need to take them, a heart-healthy diet and regular exercise may allow you to lower your dose, and thereby reduce your risk of side effects. To reverse statin-induced muscle and joint pain, try supplementing with 100 milligrams daily of the softgel form of CoQ10. For best absorption, take it with a meal containing some fat.

Avoid the Drawbacks of Antihypertensives

Blood pressure–lowering medicines carry a range of side effects. One class of drugs, diuretics (such as hydrochlorothiazide), can deplete the body of potassium, magnesium, zinc, B vitamins, and CoQ10. Ironically, potassium and magnesium are critical for keeping your blood pressure in check, and they help muscles—including your heart—work properly. Zinc helps heal wounds and boosts your immune system, B vitamins keep homocysteine levels low (▶ **49**), and CoQ10 has numerous heart benefits.

Another class called beta-blockers can cause depression, insomnia, cold extremities, fatigue, a slow heartbeat, and aggravated asthma symptoms. A 2010 study in the journal *Hypertension* found that people with abdominal obesity taking diuretics or beta-blockers, separately or together, had impaired glucose metabolism, putting them at risk for diabetes. And both classes of drugs have been linked to sexual side effects (▶ **73**).

If you're taking diuretics, restore depleted nutrients by eating potassium-rich foods such as bananas and legumes, and take 600 milligrams of magnesium, 25 to 50 milligrams of zinc, and 60 to 90 milligrams of CoQ10 daily (plus, see the B vitamin recommendations at right). If you're on beta-blockers, talk to your doctor about adjusting your dose to reduce side effects, or switch to another drug. And if you're taking any antihypertensive, eat a low-sugar, heart-healthy diet and exercise regularly to prevent diabetes (▶ **55**).

Minimize the Downside of Antidiabetes Drugs

Diabetes dramatically increases your risk of heart problems, so medications to control blood sugar, such as biguanides (Metformin), are an important part of treatment. But these drugs have the sneaky side effect of reducing levels of vitamins B6, B12, and folic acid. B vitamins support your nervous system, adrenal function, and metabolism. And shortages increase homocysteine levels, which raises your risk of kidney and heart disease and possibly Alzheimer's. Another class of drugs, thiazolidinediones, may decrease bone mineral density, and a class called alpha-glucosidase inhibitors is linked to gastrointestinal side effects, notes a 2009 study in the *American Journal of Geriatric Pharmacotherapy*.

Many daily multivitamins contain B vitamins at levels high enough to counteract the effects of antidiabetes drugs. If your multi doesn't have them, take a B-50 complex supplement with 400 micrograms of folic acid. Talk to your doctor about whether lifestyle changes can allow you to reduce your dose, or if you should switch to a different drug.

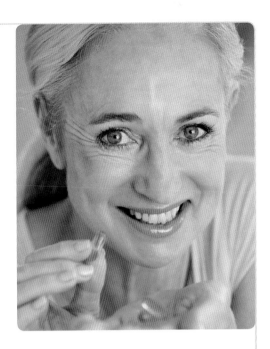

The Takeaway: Heart-Harmful Side Effects

Cholesterol-lowering statins can accelerate cardiovascular aging, in addition to causing headaches, digestive distress, and joint and muscle pain.

Diuretics, used to lower blood pressure, deplete potassium, magnesium, zinc, B vitamins, and CoQ10, which benefit the heart. If you take a diuretic, you may need to supplement to restore these lost nutrients.

Antidiabetes drugs are important for heart health if you have diabetes, but they reduce levels of B6, B12, and folic acid. If you take diabetes medications, supplement with B vitamins to regulate your nervous system, adrenal function, and metabolism.

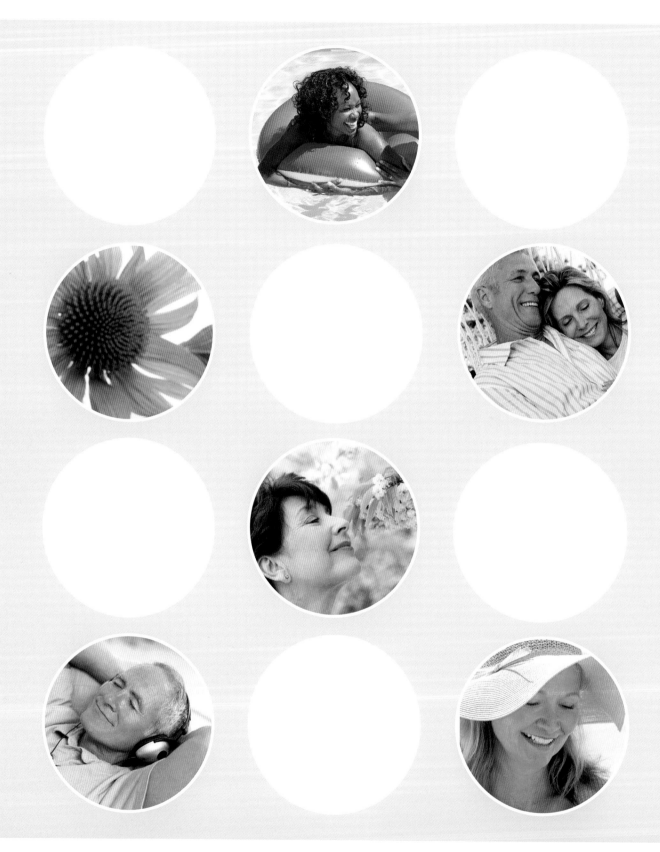

PART VI

Turn Back the Clock on Your Immune System

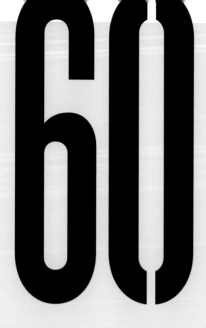

60

Let Go of a Grudge for a Younger Immune System

Over the years, your immune system gradually begins to decline. But certain lifestyle factors can hasten or delay that downturn, affecting your likelihood of staying healthy into late life. Although it's probably not the first thing you think of in terms of preserving your immunity, forgiveness is actually critical to maintaining good health for the long haul. First, it relieves stress, which suppresses your immune system, speeding its natural slowdown and leaving you more vulnerable to illness and disease as you get older (▶ 61). Second, forgiveness is essential for healthy relationships, and a strong social network acts as a further buffer to the harmful, age-accelerating effects of stress and depression (▶ 29, 57, 64).

Nursing a longstanding grudge is inherently nerve-racking, and it perpetuates stress's adverse effects far beyond the original incident. That means, ultimately, it's damaging you more than it's punishing the person who wronged you. If you can begin the process of forgiveness, however, either by finding ways to empathize or being able to genuinely wish the offender well while letting go of hurt and angry emotions, you not only neutralize the damage of unforgiving responses, but you actually cultivate positive emotional responses in their place. Called "positive affect," those responses are linked to better health overall—including a stronger immune system, according to a 2003 study by University of Wisconsin researchers. Other research indicates that forgiveness can help you sleep better at night, while anger, depression, and anxiety stemming from unforgiveness lead to poorer sleep quality, according to a 2008 study in the *Journal of Behavioral Medicine*. Getting enough rest keeps your immune system in tip-top shape and helps prevent illness as you get older (▶ 63).

Wipe the Slate Clean for a Healthier Future

You can accumulate a lot of hurts by the time you reach mid- and late life. Letting resentment fester for years, however, will weaken your immunity and set you up for health problems down the road. Before you mechanically pardon everyone on your blacklist, however, you should keep in mind a few important distinctions. Deciding to forgive someone is not the same as emotionally forgiving someone, according to a 2007 study in the *Journal of Behavioral Medicine*. The authors note that decisional forgiveness, or controlling your behavior, might reduce outward hostility, but it doesn't switch off the stress response that ultimately wears down your immunity. On the other hand, emotional forgiveness—changing your thinking, emotion, and motivation (which ultimately leads to changed behavior)—has more direct health benefits because it helps you move from a place of negativity and stress to a more hopeful, positive attitude. And staying in that happier frame of mind bolsters your immune system (▶ 65).

Cultivate Forgivingness for Lifelong Well-Being

Perhaps even more important than letting someone off the hook for a specific offense is developing what researchers call a disposition of forgivingness, which means making it a habit to extend grace to yourself and others. Highly forgiving individuals showed less depression and stress and greater subjective and psychological well-being than their less forgiving peers, according to a 2006 study in the journal *Personality and Individual Differences*. They also were more likely to engage in healthy behaviors, have strong social support, and highly rate their religious and existential spiritual well-being, all of which also tie in to better health and improved immunity.

Keep your immune system in fighting shape for years to come by choosing to forgive quickly and often. Whether you're trying to let go of a thoughtless slight or a deep wound, it's important to remember that forgiveness is a process. If you can take the first steps toward making peace, you'll usually find that

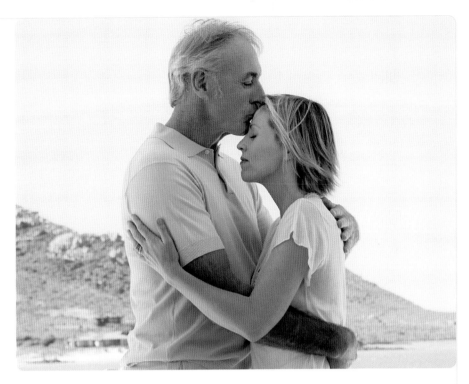

the rest will come with time. Forgiveness doesn't mean that you're saying what happened didn't matter, or that you're condoning bad behavior, either. Rather, you are refusing to let bitterness take hold and harm your health. In fact, middle-aged and older adults who showed higher levels of forgiveness toward others reported better physical and mental health, according to a 2001 study in the *Journal of Adult Development*. Forgiveness takes you out of the victim's role, puts you back in control, and frees your immune system to function at its best for a long, healthy life.

The Takeaway: Forgiveness

Let go of grudges that cause you stress; they harm you more than they affect the people you resent.

Develop a disposition of "forgivingness," pardoning quickly and often. Extend grace to others—and to yourself—and one reward will be a stronger immune system.

61

Use Mind-Body Techniques to Stop Aging Stress

Aging affects your immune system in several ways. By the time you reach sixty, your thymus gland has mostly stopped producing T cells, which are critical to immunity. That means your body has to depend on the T cells you've already stored up, and as those cells gradually change and die off, you're less able to make antibodies and your immune system doesn't "remember" past illnesses as well. (That "memory" is why you normally don't get infected with the same strain of a cold virus a second time.) Additionally, a 2008 study in the journal *Neuroimmunomodulation* found that as you get older, your immune cells—especially white blood cells—are fighting off more inflammatory compounds and free radicals with fewer antioxidant defenses to draw from. By itself, that's enough to raise your risk of infection (such as flu and pneumonia), cancer,

and autoimmune diseases as you age. But chronic stress adds an extra burden, suppressing your immune system and wearing it down even faster.

Short-term stress can actually boost your immune system, sending it into overdrive to protect you from infection and disease. But chronically elevated levels of stress hormones like cortisol and adrenaline put you in a constantly heightened state of arousal and inflammation that damages your body over time and makes your immune system less able to respond to signals to turn off that inflammation. To keep your immune system strong and healthy as you get older, managing chronic stress is crucial. You may not be able to change the source of your stress, but by taking time for yourself you can change your response to anxiety-inducing situations. Try these proven stress busters to start.

Boost Your Immunity by Doing Something You Enjoy

One smart strategy: Make it a point to pursue hobbies. People who participate in a variety of fun activities in their leisure time have reduced cortisol levels, along with several other indicators of good health, according to a 2009 study in *Psychosomatic Medicine*.

Whether it's your daily walk or a stretching session, exercise can be important "me" time. A mindfulness-based stress reduction program of twenty minutes of meditative breathing and stretching per day was enough to lower workers' stress levels by nearly 10 percent, according to a 2009 study in the journal *Health Education & Behavior*. And moderate exercise boosts immunity as well (▶**66**).

Even small acts of self-care can reduce stress. If you're stuck at the office or your home, surround yourself with calming scents to strengthen your immune system. Study participants who sniffed lavender or rosemary essential oils for five minutes lowered cortisol levels and increased their bodies' abilities to fight off aging free radicals, according to a 2007 study in the journal *Psychiatry Research*. If you can, bring in a few sprigs of fresh lavender or a potted rosemary plant—exposing yourself to nature even in small doses can snuff out stress. For example, Japanese researchers found that volunteers who stayed in a hospital room decorated with natural materials had 20 percent lower cortisol levels than those who stayed in a typical hospital room.

Laugh Often to Lighten Stress and Keep Yourself Young

Laughter not only makes you feel good, but it boosts your immune system as well, and researchers believe that the benefit stems from stress reduction. In a study published in *Alternative Therapies in Health and Medicine*, researchers asked fifty-two healthy men to watch a comedy video. After that one hour of laughing, several markers of immune function increased for up to twelve hours afterward. Further research shows that exposure to a humorous stimulus or the act of laughing can increase the activity and number of natural killer cells in the immune system. And a few small studies demonstrate an increase in salivary IgA levels (a measure of immune function) following exposure to a humorous video.

Even anticipating laughter can reduce stress and improve immunity, according to research presented at the 2008 Annual Meeting of the American Physiological Society. The study authors measured the hormones of volunteers who expected to watch a funny film, and they found that feel-good endorphins and human growth hormone (HGH), which helps with immunity, increased by 27 and 87 percent, respectively. They also found reductions in three stress hormones, including cortisol.

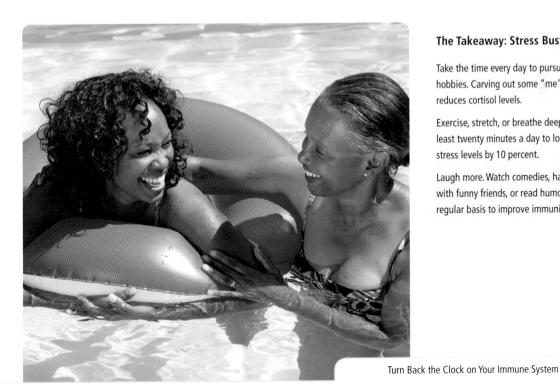

The Takeaway: Stress Busters

Take the time every day to pursue your hobbies. Carving out some "me" time reduces cortisol levels.

Exercise, stretch, or breathe deeply for at least twenty minutes a day to lower your stress levels by 10 percent.

Laugh more. Watch comedies, hang out with funny friends, or read humor on a regular basis to improve immunity.

62

Listen to Music to Restore Fading Immune Function

As you get older, your immune system grows less responsive and doesn't communicate as well with your nervous system. That means, for example, that your white blood cells can't read signals from your nervous system to turn off inflammation. Music seems able to reestablish that communication and bring hormone and neurotransmitter levels back into balance, helping your immune system function like it did when you were younger. A 2007 study in the journal *Critical Care Medicine* found that patients who listened to relaxing music for an hour had higher levels of human growth hormone, which is involved in immune function and typically declines with age. At the same time, interleukin-6 (an inflammatory compound produced by your immune system) and the stress hormone adrenaline decreased, calming inflammation and restoring healthy immune function.

In fact, much of music's ability to strengthen your immune system stems from its stress-counteracting effects. And both listening to and making music offer benefits for stress levels and immunity. After an hour of making music, volunteers over the age of sixty-five showed small increases in several markers of immune function that chronic stress typically lowers, reported researchers in a 2009 study in the *Journal of Medical and Dental Sciences*. So go ahead and whistle while you work—you might just make your immune system younger!

Music Lowers Age-Accelerating Cortisol Levels

Listening to music you enjoy can boost your mood, enhance memory and focus, and encourage you to exercise harder, and growing research shows it can also keep you calm. Besides controlling chronic stress, music can help you deal with and recover from isolated stressful events more quickly. For example, patients who were allowed to choose the kind of music they listened to during and after surgery had lowered cortisol levels and increased immunity, according to a 2007 study in the *British Journal of Surgery*. And a group of writers in a newspaper's newsroom—a classic high-stress work environment—had lowered cortisol levels after listening to music for thirty minutes while they worked, according to a study in *Psychological Reports*. For the best stress-busting benefits, pick relaxing music with a slow tempo (unless you're exercising for stress relief, in which case faster songs can give you an extra energy boost).

A caveat: Keep the volume down to avoid damaging your hearing and actually increasing your stress. A 2009

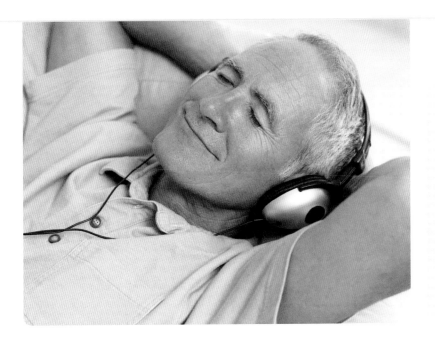

The Takeaway: Soothing Music

Listen to your favorite music during nerve-racking situations (or to calm down afterward) to reduce your stress levels.

Make music to stimulate your mind and body while boosting immunity.

Sing in a choir or join a jam band to get the dual benefits of music and social interaction.

study in the journal *Environmental Health Perspectives* found that women who were exposed to noise louder than 60 decibels had cortisol levels 34 percent higher than those who listened to noise at 50 decibels or less. To protect your hearing, turn the volume on your stereo down a notch or two, and limit using in-ear headphones, or earbuds, to a few hours a day at 70 percent volume or less.

Make Your Own Music to Improve Your Immunity

In addition to listening to your favorite tunes, making music also reduces stress and keeps your immune system functioning optimally as you get older. A 2005 study in the journal *Medical Science Monitor* found that people who participated in a recreational music-making activity after being exposed to a stressful situation significantly lowered several markers of the stress

response compared to those who just rested. In fact, making music may have a stress-soothing edge over other relaxing activities. Japanese researchers found that employees who made music for an hour had lower levels of stress-induced inflammation and increased natural killer cell activity (a marker of immune function) than those who read leisurely.

Whether you enjoy the communal experience of singing in a choir or the physicality of banging on bongos, making music with others can offer mental, social, and physical stimulation (a combination that's also key to boosting your brainpower as you get older [▶33]). That can further increase the stress-reduction benefits, since mixing those elements engages your mind and your body to change your stress response. If you don't want to join a musical group, try gathering friends to

play a video game like Rock Band. But you don't have to go public with your musical talents to keep your immune system young: Solo music making still counts. Sing in the shower or the car, or drum on your desk while you're waiting for Web pages to load.

63

Don't Skimp on Sleep As You Get Older

While you're sleeping, your body is busy repairing itself. When you don't get enough sleep, or don't sleep deeply, that healing doesn't happen as well. That can spell big trouble for your immune system as you get older, putting you at increased risk of infection and disease. In a healthy brain, substances related to immunity interact with neurochemical systems to regulate your sleep. But as you age, communication between your immune system and your nervous system begins to break down. A lack of sleep can further upset the balance, aging your immune system so it can't protect you as well.

Researchers don't know exactly how sleep impacts immunity, but some suspect that your body's circadian rhythms affect immune system cells, or that sleep may reduce immunity-weakening oxidative stress (in effect, functioning as an anti-aging free-radical fighter). The sleep-regulating hormone melatonin, which also decreases with age, influences several aspects of immunity as well. In fact, researchers are currently investigating whether supplementing with melatonin can restore immune function in older people.

You need at least seven hours a night to reach healing REM sleep, evidence indicates. A 2009 study in the *Archives of Internal Medicine* found that volunteers who got less than seven hours of sleep nightly for two weeks were nearly three times as likely to develop a cold when exposed to a virus. Thankfully, putting the following sleep habits into practice may be enough to restore that nightly healing process and keep your immune system functioning at its best as you get older.

Smart Strategies to Help You Sleep like a Baby

In later life, many people don't sleep as well as they used to, thanks to medications, hormonal shifts, changing responsibilities, and chronic conditions. For example, common drugs like beta-blockers for high blood pressure and nonsteroidal anti-inflammatory drugs (NSAIDs) for joint pain significantly lower melatonin production, thereby aggravating insomnia. If you have trouble sleeping, keeping a sleep journal in which you record activities, what you eat and drink, how you feel, or other factors that influence how well you sleep may shed some light on what's interfering with a good night's rest. If your sleep problems last longer than two weeks, talk to your doctor about possible underlying factors.

Some basic steps you can take to set the stage for sleep include reserving your bed (and ideally your bedroom) for sleeping and sex, avoiding stimulating activities before bed, and sticking to a regular sleep schedule (▶19, 32). Exercise regularly, but not in the few hours before you go to bed. And if anxiety keeps you awake at night, try pouring out your thoughts in a journal or make a to-do list so you don't keep ruminating.

To minimize sleep interruptions and ensure you get enough immune-boosting REM sleep, keep your bedroom completely dark and quiet, don't consume caffeine or alcohol for several hours before bedtime (if you're sensitive, you may need to cut them out completely), and limit nighttime beverages. Napping to make up for lost Zzzs may actually make it harder to fall and stay asleep at night, when the immune system needs it most, so keep daytime snoozing to a minimum if possible.

Try Natural Remedies to Sleep Better As You Age

If you try these approaches and still have trouble falling asleep, have a few sips of chamomile tea or warm milk before bed. Both have relaxing properties, and having something warm in your stomach can be comforting. Two of the best natural sleep aids are valerian (*Valeriana officinalis*) and melatonin. Valerian, an herbal sedative that's been used for centuries, is nontoxic and not addictive, but some people find it leaves them feeling fuzzy-headed in the morning. If you'd like to try it, take one or two capsules of a product standardized to 1 percent valerenic acid thirty minutes before bedtime.

Supplemental melatonin is also available over the counter. Other than causing an increase in dreaming, it has no known side effects. Andrew Weil, M.D., an integrative physician, author, and professor, recommends taking 2.5 milligrams at bedtime occasionally if needed. He prefers sublingual tablets that dissolve when you place them under the tongue, but capsules are also an option. For regular use, a much lower dose (0.25 to 0.3 milligrams) may be effective.

The Takeaway: Sleep Soundly

Keep a journal to determine if your diet, exercise routines, anxiety over a personal issue, or other factors are at the root of your sleeping problems.

Reserve your bedroom for sleeping and sex and keep it dark and quiet.

Exercise regularly, but avoid working out and doing other stimulating activities before bedtime. Instead, soothe yourself by drinking warm tea or milk.

If you still aren't sleeping well, try taking valerian or melatonin.

64

Use the Power of Touch for Lifelong Immunity

Your hardworking immune system naturally slows down as you get older, leaving it less responsive and able to protect you from infection and disease. But science reveals several strategies for shoring up your immune system, including touch, whether from a friendly hug, a massage, or even sex.

Much of the research on how touch improves immunity has focused on massage therapy in people with cancer or HIV/AIDS. But as the evidence becomes more convincing, researchers are branching out to explore how other forms of touch can benefit people with reduced immunity, such as late-life adults. For example, Japanese researchers found that for older patients who were bedridden after having a stroke, giving their skin a light rubdown with a dry towel for ten minutes a day increased natural killer cell activity.

Massage improves several markers of immune function, such as lymphocyte, T cell, and natural killer cell counts, according to a 2010 review of studies. Researchers suspect much of the benefit comes from stress reduction (the stress hormone cortisol, for example, destroys natural killer cells—the immune system's front line of defense), and science seems to bear that out. Massage therapy lowers immune-suppressing cortisol levels by an average of 31 percent, according to a 2005 review of studies in the *International Journal of Neuroscience*. At the same time, massage increases the feel-good neurotransmitters dopamine and serotonin, helping prevent or lift depression. Since depression is linked to decreased cellular immunity (▶65), that's a significant benefit.

The social contact involved also seems to play a role: A 2003 study in the journal *Psychological Science* found that the more social people are, the less likely they are to develop a cold when exposed to a cold virus. (There aren't many studies on the benefits of self-massage, such as a foot rubdown or hand massage, but what evidence there is indicates that it may also reduce anxiety and boost mood.)

Give a Hug, Get a Hug to Ward Off Illness

Offer new acquaintances a handshake, hug your friends, hold hands with your romantic partner or request a neck rub when you're tense—all of these forms of touch not only promote feelings of social connection, but they can help bolster a weakening immune system as you get older. One of the ways touching another person, even briefly, can help is by soothing stress. For example, holding hands can reduce anxiety in a stressful situation, reports a 2001 study in the *Journal of Advanced Nursing*.

Supportive social relationships also seem to buffer the effects of stress on immunity, thereby allowing an aging immune system to function better (▶**61**). Research shows that massage (and, by extension, other forms of touch) and social interaction both spur production of oxytocin, a hormone made in the brain that stimulates our desire to connect with others. It can increase feelings of trust, generosity, and love, and studies show it also lowers cortisol levels and several markers of inflammation, potentially helping a declining immune system keep inflammation levels in check.

Have Sex for a Stronger Immune System

Physical intimacy often wanes as you get older, but a good sexual relationship may provide significant immunity-strengthening benefits, such as reducing stress and helping you sleep better. And it can boost levels of important immune system markers: A 2004 study in the journal *Psychological Reports* found that men and women who had sex once or twice a week had higher levels of an immune system protein called immunoglobulin A (IgA) than those who had less sex. Your body also produces sky-high levels of oxytocin during orgasm, which bolsters your immunity and fosters feelings of closeness.

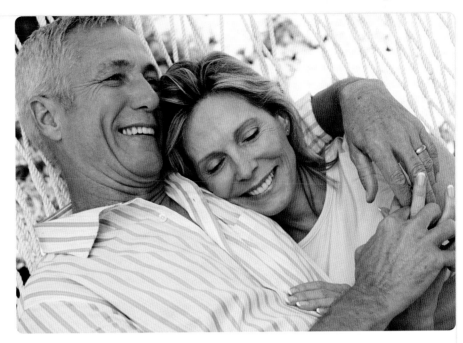

Around age sixty, your thymus gland mostly stops producing new T cells critical to a healthy immune system (▶**61**). However, your skin secretes a similar immune hormone, and it just needs a little stimulation to step up production and offset the aging of the thymus. Sex triggers the biggest release, but other forms of touch such as back rubs and snuggling can also signal your skin to secrete this immune-strengthening hormone.

The Takeaway: Touch for Health

Hug friends and hold hands with loved ones to boost feelings of well-being.

Get a massage to soothe stress and activate immunity-boosting hormones.

Have sex or embrace your lover to produce high levels of immunity-strengthening oxytocin.

65

Look on the Bright Side to Reduce Immune System Decline

A positive outlook confers many health benefits, including lower blood pressure and better recovery from surgery. And research shows it can also improve immunity, both by mediating immune-suppressing stress and actively boosting several markers of a healthy immune system. For older adults, the difference may even be significant enough to offset the natural decline of their immune systems.

A generally sunny disposition, as well as having specific high hopes, seems to buffer the damaging effects of stress on the immune system (▶61). For instance, people characterized as being anxious, hostile, and depressed were three times more likely to get sick when exposed to a cold or flu virus than their happy, lively, and calm counterparts, noted a 2006 study in *Psychosomatic Medicine*. Feeling like you have control over your circumstances makes a difference too.

When study participants had actual or perceived control over a stressor, the optimists had better natural killer cell function than their pessimistic peers, reports a 2005 study in the journal *Brain, Behavior, and Immunity*.

In another study where participants received a vaccine, optimism protected against the inflammatory effects of stress. Perhaps even more important, however, the optimistic volunteers had a higher antibody response to the vaccine. During a similar study, researchers at the University of Pittsburgh found that people with what's scientifically called "positive affect" (broadly defined as feelings that reflect pleasurable engagement with the environment) responded better to a hepatitis vaccination than people who were negative, moody, nervous, and easily stressed. Since one of the main signs of an aging immune system is being less responsive to vaccinations, these results are very good news for anyone hoping to keep their immune system young and healthy.

Cultivate Optimism for a Stronger Immune System

Evidence indicates that optimism can be learned. "Optimism is not only a matter of perspective, it's also a matter of choice," points out Jason F. Mathers, Ph.D., a licensed psychologist in private practice. So how do you become more positive if you don't naturally have an upbeat outlook? "In working with my clients," says Mathers, "I often challenge their negative thought patterns by teaching them a four-step process of confrontation, consisting of: a) recognizing the negative thought patterns; b) labeling the thoughts as detrimental to their well-being; c) identifying positive alternatives; and d) making a concerted effort to replace the negative thoughts with the alternatives." And since optimists do better than pessimists in almost every aspect of life—including immunity—experts agree it's worth making the effort.

Surrounding yourself with cheerful people can also help you change your perspective. If you're having trouble breaking out of negative thought patterns, you might even ask a particularly positive friend how she might see your situation in a better light. Funny friends who can help you laugh, at yourself or your circumstances, are also worth seeking out. Laughter boosts your mood, making it easier for you to focus on positive thoughts, and it also relieves stress that can further weaken an aging immune system (▶61).

Put a Stop to Immunity-Sapping Pessimism

Studies have shown that a positive mood is associated with stronger cellular immunity. On the flip side, a 2009 study in the journal *Brain, Behavior, and Immunity* found that pessimism actually accelerated aging and weakened immune function in postmenopausal women. Making an effort to be more positive may also protect you against depression down the road. "More than once I've seen optimism be the only thing that stands between a person falling into a full-blown depression and that same person thriving in the face of adversity," says Mathers.

Depression, which is linked to feelings of hopelessness and pessimism, can be harmful to health. For starters, people who are depressed generally don't exercise as much, sleep as well, or eat as healthfully—neglecting the building blocks of immunity. Depression also triggers inflammation and suppresses natural killer cell activity and the creation of T cells that fight off infection.

Pessimism is contagious, so minimize the time you spend with complainers, cynics, and other negative people. Talk to your doctor if you suspect you're depressed. And don't let pessimism make you passive: "An optimistic person takes hold of the possibility of a [positive] outcome and often works or even fights to make that happen," notes Mathers.

The Takeaway: Choose Optimism

Recognize that negative thought patterns are harmful to your health; identify positive alternatives and work to change your thinking.

Surround yourself with optimistic people and friends who make you laugh.

Avoid pessimists; their dour attitudes can be contagious.

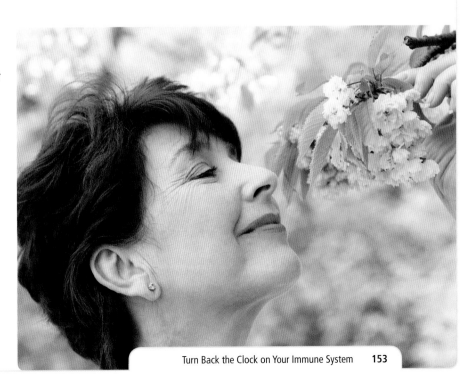

66

Exercise in Moderation to Maintain Immunity As You Age

While strength training, balance, and flexibility exercises are critical for slowing down the aging process and keeping you young and healthy, studies show that aerobic exercise offers the most immune-boosting effects. Exercise can help shore up your immune system in the short term and over the long haul, providing extra protection against infection and disease as your body's natural defenses begin to decline. For instance, immediately after a group of women completed a thirty-minute walking workout, researchers noted that several measures of their immune function improved, including increased counts of germ-fighting white blood cells and natural killer cells and reduced markers of inflammation, according to a 2005 study in *Medicine and Science in Sports and Exercise*.

Several studies have shown that working out regularly provides ongoing support for the immune system as well, including a 2005 study in the journal *Neuroendocrinology Letters* that found consistent, moderate exercise increases levels of immunoglobulins, antibodies in your blood that fight off illness. And other research indicates that exercise increases the effectiveness of vaccines, which is increasingly important as you get older, since an aging immune system is less responsive to vaccination. Previously sedentary older adults who exercised regularly after they received a flu shot showed a significant increase in vaccine-related protection against the flu as much as twenty-four weeks later, according to a 2009 study in the *Journal of the American Geriatrics Society*. Not only that, but they also slept better and, when they did get sick, had less severe respiratory tract infections than nonexercisers throughout the entire cold and flu season.

Research shows that thirty to forty-five minutes of moderate exercise on most days of the week will strengthen your immune defenses. A 2006 study in the *American Journal of Medicine* found that women who did forty-five minutes of moderate-intensity exercise five days per week for a year had increasingly improved immunity, to the point that by the end of the study they were three times less likely to catch a cold than those assigned to forty-five minutes of once-weekly stretching sessions.

The calories you burn through aerobic exercise also help you stave off obesity, which reduces immunity by aging the thymus system and slowing its production of T cells, a type of white blood cell. In addition, regular exercise helps you sleep better (▶**63**) and may even motivate you to eat healthfully (▶**67**), both of which help keep your immune system young and strong.

Overdoing Exercise Can Age Your Immune System

Adding high-intensity intervals to your exercise routine can help you increase speed and endurance and burn more calories in less time (▶**94**). However, research shows that this and other intense or prolonged exercise, such as training for a race, can actually suppress your immune system. For example, a 2008 review of studies in the *Clinical Journal of Sports Medicine* noted that particularly strenuous exercise may diminish activity of natural killer cells. A 2007 study in the *European Journal of Applied Physiology* found that high-intensity sessions can decrease neutrophils, a kind of white blood cell, and raise levels of interleukin-6, a marker of inflammation. You'll see the most dramatic decline in immunity when exercise is continuous, prolonged, of moderate to high intensity, and performed without eating or drinking, noted U.K. researchers in a 2006 study.

But that doesn't mean you should avoid high-intensity training if you enjoy it, experts say. Eating healthfully (including plenty of protein and carbohydrates), plus maintaining other immune-supporting habits such as getting enough sleep and managing stress go a long way to keeping you healthy and infection-free. If you exercise for more than ninety minutes, be sure to consume carbohydrates (such as a sports drink) during your workout to counteract the rise in stress hormones and minimize immune system suppression, suggests a 2008 study in *Nutrition Reviews*. The researchers also note that supplementing with antioxidants such as quercetin (a plant compound found in tea, fruits, and vegetables) and curcumin (a component of the curry spice turmeric) might help counteract the stress of strenuous exercise and restore white blood cell function. A small study reported immunity improvements in endurance cyclists taking 1,000 milligrams of quercetin supplements daily for three weeks before and during long bouts of exercise. More research is needed to determine the best postexercise dose of curcumin, though regular dietary intake may be enough—even small amounts show antioxidant action and other benefits (▶**26**).

The Takeaway: Exercise in Moderation

Aerobic exercise is best for boosting immunity; try to do thirty to forty-five minutes at moderate intensity five days a week.

High-intensity exercise actually dampens the immune response, leaving you vulnerable to catching colds and other viruses.

If you exercise for more than ninety minutes, consume carbohydrates (such as a sports drink) or supplement with quercetin or curcumin to counteract the increased stress and restore white blood cell function.

61

Supercharge Your Diet with Immune-Boosting Foods

Free radicals accelerate aging throughout the body, and your immune system is no exception. In fact, research shows that your immune system, especially your white blood cells, faces increasing amounts of free radicals as you get older. Fighting off that oxidative damage with antioxidants, therefore, is a surefire strategy to keep your immune system young and strong. Antioxidant vitamins, minerals, and nutrients protect and repair immune system cells, improving your body's ability to defend itself against colds, flus, and other infections. Research shows that several other foods offer protective compounds as well, and they all fit into a healthy diet—even antioxidant-rich dark chocolate! In general, your body absorbs nutrients better from foods than from supplements, so round out your diet with these superfoods and you'll be well on your way to super immunity.

Slow Aging with Antioxidant-Rich Fruits and Vegetables

An abundance of antioxidants such as the B vitamins, vitamins C and E, beta-carotene, and compounds called flavonoids make fruits and vegetables immune-strengthening powerhouses. Aim for five to nine servings per day, and eat a variety of different-colored produce to ensure you get a good mix of all the anti-aging antioxidants they offer. For example, orange-hued sweet potatoes and carrots contain vitamin C and beta-carotene, blue and red berries boast anthocyanins and other flavonoids, and bright red watermelon provides the powerful antioxidant glutathione. For the best free radical–scavenging benefits, eat these foods raw or lightly steamed (overcooking can destroy the antioxidants, and boiling leaches nutrients into the cooking water).

Broccoli and other cruciferous vegetables such as cabbage contain glutathione and the antioxidant compound sulforaphane. When researchers treated older mice with sulforaphane, the compound increased their immune response to the level of younger mice, according to a 2008 study in the *Journal of Allergy and Clinical Immunology*.

Mushrooms offer a few particular benefits as well. Asian mushrooms (shiitake, maitake) contain beta-glucans, a type of carbohydrate that boosts the immune system. And regular old button mushrooms provide antioxidants such as selenium as well as the B vitamins riboflavin and niacin; riboflavin increases resistance to bacterial infections, while niacin reduces oxidative stress and inflammation. Lab and animal studies also indicate mushrooms have antiviral, antibacterial, and antitumor effects.

Garlic gets its odor from the sulfur compound allicin, which also increases the production of white blood cells. In addition, a 2007 study in the *Journal of Interferon & Cytokine Research* found that eating 2 grams (less than a teaspoon) of fresh garlic stimulated the production of nitric oxide and interferonalpha, which activate immune cells and help fight viral infections. Fresh garlic seems to be best, but if you don't like the taste, peel, chop, and let it sit fifteen to twenty minutes before gently cooking to activate immune-boosting enzymes.

Eat a Daily Serving of Other Immune-Boosting Foods

White, green, and black tea are some of the healthiest drinks around, offering vitamin C and antioxidant flavonoids and polyphenols. (Caffeinated and decaf varieties work equally well.) Nuts also provide antioxidant vitamins and minerals. Almonds, for example, offer nearly 50 percent of the recommended daily amount of vitamin E per quarter-cup serving. They also boast the B vitamins riboflavin and niacin. Brazil nuts provide exceptional amounts of selenium (one nut contains almost 100 micrograms, or nearly twice the recommended daily amount). A 2008 review of studies noted that selenium supports the immune system in several ways, partly by offsetting the effects of aging on immunity.

Red meat also serves up selenium and the immune-boosting mineral zinc. Zinc speeds wound healing and may have an antiviral effect as well. Low levels of zinc impair immunity, decrease resistance to germs, and are linked to more frequent and severe bouts of pneumonia in older adults (and, as a result, longer rounds of treatment), noted a 2010 study in *Nutrition Reviews*. Oysters and wheat germ are also good sources.

Probiotics, or "good" bacteria, may spur your immune system to fight disease. They're especially beneficial if you've been taking antibiotics, which wipe out all bacteria—good and bad—in your system. That can compromise your immune response—specifically, the function of white blood cells called neutrophils, suggests a 2007 study in *Nature Medicine*. Yogurt with live and active cultures is a prime source, but more and more foods are being fortified with these friendly bacteria.

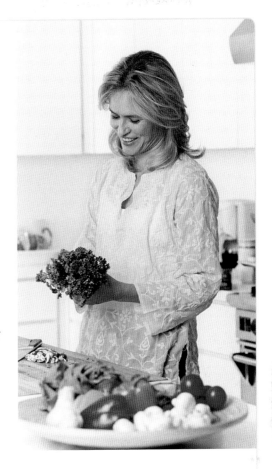

The Takeaway: Foods for Super Immunity

Eat a rainbow of colorful fruits and vegetables to reap anti-aging antioxidants.

Mushrooms and garlic will help you fight off viral infections and other illnesses.

Have a serving of nuts or a little red meat for minerals that boost immunity.

Drink white, green, or black tea (caffeinated or decaf) for a dose of vitamin C and antioxidants.

68

Take Herbs That Support an Aging Immune System

In addition to getting enough rest, exercising regularly, and eating plenty of antioxidant-rich foods—the building blocks of healthy immunity—you may want to consider taking an herbal supplement to counteract the natural decline in your immune system as you get older. However, it's important to remember that a pill can't make up for an unhealthy lifestyle, and just because these herbs are natural doesn't mean they're automatically safe for you to take. Read labels carefully and obey warnings, and let your doctor know you'd like to try them, since some herbs can interact with drugs or other natural remedies.

Prevent Immune System Decline with North American Ginseng

The antioxidant and anti-inflammatory herb North American ginseng (*Panax quinquefolius*) contains compounds called ginsenosides and polysaccharides that seem to be responsible for the herb's immune-boosting effects. It broadly supports the immune system and protects against stress, and you can take it indefinitely to help shore up your immune system as it naturally slows down with age. A 2009 review of studies in *Evidence-Based Complementary and Alternative Medicine* concluded that while North American ginseng doesn't reliably reduce the incidence or severity of colds and respiratory infections, it appears to shorten their duration. The herb might also exert antitumor effects: A ginseng extract slowed the spread of and killed human colon cancer cells in lab tests, according to a 2010 study in *Phytomedicine*.

Preparations and quality of this herb vary widely, so look for standardized products that indicate the ginsenoside content and follow the package dosing directions. Take it regularly throughout the cold and flu season, or at the first sign of a cold to shorten its duration. If you use it long-term, take two to three weeks off every four months. People with fibroids or with a history of breast cancer shouldn't take it, and it can interact with some drugs for heart disease, diabetes, and depression.

Increase Your Immunity with Astragalus

Astragalus membranaceous is another nontoxic herb you can take indefinitely to improve disease resistance and help fight off chronic or recurrent infections. Despite its long history of use in China, it hasn't been studied often in humans. Astragalus reduced production of several inflammatory markers in mouse cells, according to a 2008 study in the *Journal of Medicinal Food*. In other lab and animal studies, astragalus increased

T cell counts in samples with low levels (common in older adults), enhanced antibody responses, and improved white blood cells' ability to eliminate harmful intruders. Additionally, astragalus restored the white blood cell response of older mice to levels normally found in younger mice and partially reestablished immune function in mice with tumors or other immune problems, noted a 2007 study in the *Journal of Ethnopharmacology*. In one of the few human studies, patients with depressed immune systems due to stomach trauma were given astragalus, which helped restore cellular immunity. And in a pair of studies investigating astragalus, echinacea, and licorice, researchers found that each of the supplements boosted immune cell activity for up to seven days (the combination was even more powerful).

Look for standardized extracts of astragalus in liquid, capsule, or tablet form. Follow the daily dosing directions on the package. People who are on immune-suppressing drugs to treat cancer or who are organ-transplant recipients should not use astragalus.

Shorten the Duration of Colds with Echinacea

Also called purple coneflower, echinacea (*E. purpurea* and *E. angustifolia*) is one of the most-studied herbs for cold prevention. Lab and animal studies indicate it has antiviral and anti-inflammatory properties and activates white blood cells. And while studies in humans show echinacea doesn't prevent colds, it does seem to shorten their duration. A 2007 study in the *International Journal of Sports Medicine* noted that volunteers who took echinacea for four weeks had higher levels of antibodies, and in those who caught respiratory infections, symptoms lasted less than half as long as in those taking a placebo (about 3.4 days, compared to 8.6 days).

Buy products that contain both purpurea and angustifolia species standardized to 4 percent echinacosides. Take echinacea at the first sign of a cold, but don't use it continuously for more than ten days. Take one dropperful of tincture in water four times a day, or two capsules of freeze-dried extract four times a day, or follow the package directions. Don't use echinacea if you have an autoimmune condition such as lupus or rheumatoid arthritis.

The Takeaway: Powerful Herbs

Take North American ginseng indefinitely to boost immunity and shorten the duration of colds.

Try astragalus, long used in China, to improve disease resistance and fight chronic infections.

Take echinacea for up to ten days to shorten the duration of upper respiratory infections.

69

Improve Your Air Quality to Avoid Aging Your Immune System

Because the immune system naturally slows down as you age, older adults are especially vulnerable to the immune-weakening effects of poor air quality. Cigarette smoke and air pollution are two of the biggest offenders, largely because they create massive amounts of free radicals. Highly reactive molecules, free radicals have one or more unpaired electrons. They scavenge healthy cells to find electrons to pair up with, damaging cells and making them vulnerable to invading viruses and germs. While some free radicals occur naturally in the body without causing problems, older people battle more free radicals than younger adults do, and they have fewer natural antioxidants with which to defend themselves. As a result, free-radical damage from poor air quality adds an extra burden to your body, ultimately aging your immune system and increasing your risk of illness.

Exposure to tobacco smoke also reduces your body's production of cytokines (immune system substances responsible for cell communication) and impairs the response of proteins that recognize invading microbes and activate the immune system. And air pollutants trigger a reaction in your immune system that causes inflammation and irritation in many people. A 2009 study in the journal *Respirology* noted that inhaling toxic particles and gases reduces your body's innate defenses by suppressing white blood cell function and triggering inflammation in your lungs and throughout your body. People who are sensitive to these substances may have especially severe reactions.

Airborne particles come from many sources, including power plants, incinerators, vehicle exhaust, wood stoves and fireplaces, and candles. Even short-term exposure to these particles—smoke, dust, dirt, soot, and liquid droplets—can aggravate asthma and existing respiratory conditions, as well as increase your susceptibility to new respiratory infections. Ozone pollution is another factor: It's linked to reduced defense against harmful bacteria, noted researchers at Duke University Medical Center, and it can worsen asthma as well. Unfortunately, indoor air quality can be just as bad as outdoor, especially if outdoor pollution levels are frequently high in your area.

Weather plays a role in air quality as well. Stagnant air or high air pressure can trap pollutants near the ground, but wind can stir up pollen and other allergens that aggravate asthma and allergies. (Pollen affects your immune system differently than pollutants—it activates antibodies that trigger histamine production and lead to inflammation.) Dry air may also make you more vulnerable to colds and flu because it irritates the mucous membranes, your trusty barriers against invading bugs.

Reduce Pollutants to Keep Your Immune System Young

Avoid exposure to air pollution as much as you can. If you exercise outdoors, choose a route with as little traffic as possible: A 2009 study in *Environmental Health Perspectives* found that postmenopausal women who exercised near roadways had 21 percent lower natural killer cell function (a measure of immunity). Also, pay attention to weather forecasts, pollution advisories, and pollen counts in your area to determine if you should limit your time outdoors.

To boost your body's defenses, increase your intake of antioxidant-rich foods, especially fresh fruits and vegetables (▶**67**). If you live in an area with poor air quality, you may want to consider taking North American ginseng or astragalus (▶**68**) to boost your overall immunity and restore some of the immune function lost due to pollution.

To improve your indoor air quality, reduce the use of candles, wood-burning stoves, and fireplaces. HEPA (high-efficiency particulate air) filters effectively remove airborne particles by forcing them through screens with

microscopic pores, and they don't generate ozone like some filters. They're also relatively inexpensive. Houseplants act as natural air filters, soaking up harmful gases and giving off oxygen. Common choices like English ivy, spider plants, golden pothos, peace lilies, and philodendrons are among the best air cleaners.

To combat dry air, use a humidifier in your bedroom at night or use a saline nasal spray occasionally to keep your mucous membranes moist. Drink plenty of water, and cut back on alcohol and caffeine, which can dehydrate you. You may also want to increase your intake of omega-3s, which can help moisturize skin and mucous membranes from the inside out (▶**3**).

The Takeaway: Breathe Cleaner Air

Cigarette smoke creates massive amounts of aging free radicals, and exposure impairs immune system activation.

Air pollution causes inflammation, irritation, and asthma in many people. Don't exercise near roadways, and pay attention to pollution advisories.

Indoors, avoid burning candles or wood in stoves and fireplaces. Consider using a HEPA filter or getting air-cleaning houseplants.

Use a humidifier and saline spray to keep mucous membranes moist.

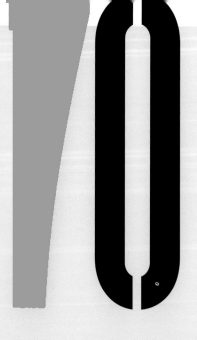

Avoid the Sniffles to Keep Your Immune System Strong for Life

It seems unfair, but as you get older and your immune system slows down, your risk of getting sick increases. Then, in the spirit of kicking you while you're down, getting an infection like bronchitis or the flu can weaken your immune system even more and increase your chances of developing a more severe illness, such as pneumonia, that takes a long time to recover from and can bring potentially deadly complications. So preventing relatively mild conditions like colds, sinus infections, or strep throat relieves stress on your immune system, allowing it to function optimally and focus on keeping heavy hitters like pneumonia, cancer, and other chronic diseases at bay.

Taking antibiotics to treat an infection or other condition can also weaken your immune system. In fact, a 2005 study in the *Archives of Dermatology* found that patients taking antibiotics long-term had twice the risk of developing upper respiratory tract infections. Antibiotics wipe out the "good" bacteria along with the bad, and upsetting the balance between the two compromises your immune response—specifically, the function of white blood cells called neutrophils, suggests a 2007 study in *Nature Medicine*.

Practice Prevention for Healthy Aging

All the tips in part VI will strengthen your natural defenses and help you ward off infections and diseases. As you get older, it's especially important to practice basic habits that keep you from getting every bug that goes around. That means washing your hands with soap and water regularly (or using an alcohol-based sanitizer if you don't have access to water), not touching your face, coughing and sneezing into a tissue or your elbow, cleaning shared surfaces like phones and keyboards frequently, and avoiding crowds during cold and flu season.

You should also get a flu shot, and make sure you're up to date on other vaccines, such as whooping cough. Only about 65 percent of older people get the flu vaccine (and as few as 30 percent of people with high-risk conditions such as diabetes and heart disease), according to the Centers for Disease Control and Prevention. Even though the annual shots don't work as well for aging immune systems as they do younger ones, they still offer critical protection and give your immune system a jump-start on fighting off the infection. Remember that an optimistic outlook (▶65) and moderate exercise (▶66) can actually improve your response to vaccines! If you do still get the flu, it will likely be milder than if you hadn't been

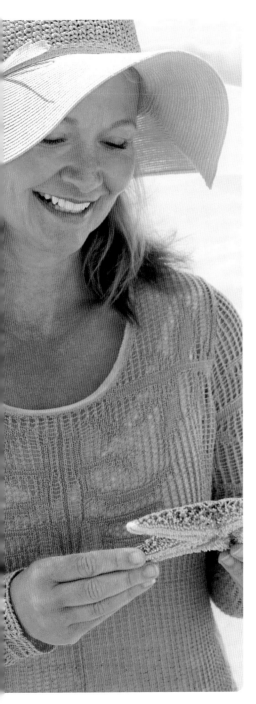

vaccinated, and therefore less likely to progress to something more dangerous.

Strategies to Strengthen Your Immune System

If you do get sick and end up with a fever, you should let it run its course. Except for certain groups of people, such as the very young and the very old, or people with certain medical conditions such as heart or lung disease, doctors no longer recommend suppressing a low-grade fever. That's because a low-grade fever actually helps your body fight off infection; a higher body temperature makes it harder for germs to grow and multiply, and it activates the immune system, helping it to respond faster to invaders. That said, if your fever has lasted more than three days, or if your temperature is more than 103°F (39°C), you should call your doctor.

Also, don't ask your doctor for antibiotics if you don't need them. Colds and flus are viral infections, for example, and won't respond to antibiotics. However, if you do have to take antibiotics, eat a cup of yogurt with live and active cultures daily until you've finished the full course and for a few days afterward to replenish immune-supporting "good" bacteria in your digestive tract. Alternatively, you can take a probiotic supplement, which contains much higher amounts of friendly bacteria. Check the expiration date, and look for products that provide billions of "colony forming units" (CFUs) and contain strains of

Bacillus coagulans, *Lactobacillus GG*, or *Bifidobacterium*. (Other strains may not survive the acidic environment of the stomach and make it to your lower GI tract, where they're needed.) Follow the package directions for dosing, and store the package in the refrigerator to protect it from heat, moisture, and air.

The Takeaway: Preventive Measures

Protect yourself against viruses by washing your hands with soap and water, avoiding crowds during cold and flu season, and getting a flu shot.

Let a low-grade fever run its course. Your body's higher temperature will kick your immune system into gear.

Don't request antibiotics for a cold or flu; they won't cure it. If you must take antibiotics, supplement with probiotic capsules or a cup of yogurt with live and active cultures until a few days after you're off the meds.

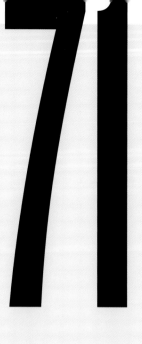

Shun the Sun to Preserve a Youthful Immune System

Americans spent more than $7 billion on anti-aging treatments for the skin in 2008, according to the American Academy of Dermatology. But your most effective anti-aging treatment might be a $5 bottle of sunscreen—and not just because it protects your skin from wrinkles and other signs of sun damage. Too much ultraviolet (UV) radiation can actually suppress your immune system. Two kinds of UV wavelengths reach the earth: ultraviolet A (UVA) and ultraviolet B (UVB). Research indicates that UVB rays increase your risk of DNA changes that can develop into skin cancer, and UVA rays create free radicals that not only damage DNA but also impair your immune system, making it less able to defend against cancerous changes and other dangerous invaders. Those free radicals speed up the aging of your immune system, hastening the natural decline of your body's defenses.

Exposure to immune-suppressing UVA rays causes a defect in the development of T cells (a type of white blood cell) that impairs their ability to become "long-term memory" cells, according to a 2010 study in the journal *Photochemical & Photobiological Sciences*. Australian researchers demonstrated that UVB rays have a similar effect. Memory cells allow your immune system to remember and defend against illnesses and bugs you've already encountered, such as chicken pox. Since your body gradually stops producing "naïve" T cells by the time you reach your mid-sixties, your immune system increasingly depends on existing memory T cells to keep you healthy as you get older.

On the other hand, sun exposure allows skin to synthesize vitamin D, which boosts immunity by affecting white blood cells' response to infection, notes a 2010 study in *Molecular and Cellular Endocrinology*. That doesn't give you a free pass to skip sunscreen, however. Experts point out that you're better off getting vitamin D from foods and supplements (▶42, 43), since as you age, your body becomes less efficient at producing vitamin D from the sun, and because the risks of sun exposure to your skin and your immune system are so high.

Boost Your Immunity with Antioxidant-Enriched Sunscreen

Since both UVA and UVB rays suppress your immune system, look for sunscreens labeled "broad spectrum" that shield you from each. Apply 1 ounce (30 ml, or the amount in a shot glass) of SPF 15 sunscreen half an hour before heading outdoors—even on hazy days, since UV rays can penetrate cloud cover. If you have fair skin or burn easily, opt for SPF 30. Reapply every two hours (▶2). No sunscreen can block all UV rays, however, so some radiation still reaches skin and creates free radicals. Adding antioxidants to your sunscreen can neutralize age-accelerating oxidative damage. A 2009 study in the *Journal of Investigative Dermatology* found that antioxidant plant compounds called polyphenols, such as epigallocatechin-3-gallate (EGCG) from green tea, protect against UV-induced DNA damage and immune suppression, thanks to their ability to quench free radicals and regulate a protein that coordinates the immune response to infection. Look for bottles combining vitamins C and E and/or EGCG with a broad-spectrum sunscreen for the most effective protection.

Trim Your Time in the Sun to Avoid Aging Free Radicals

Even better than sunscreen? Limiting your sun exposure, especially between 10 a.m. and 4 p.m., when the sun shines the strongest. Even darker-skinned people who don't burn easily should seek shade whenever possible, since UV rays penetrate skin deeply to create immunity-lowering free radicals and DNA damage even without a visible sunburn. You might also wear a hat and sun-protective clothing if you'll be outside for a while. Swap your baseball cap or golf visor for a broad-brimmed topper to shield your face and neck better. Wear tightly woven, loose-fitting, and dark-colored clothing, or purchase pieces specifically designed to offer sun protection. Such products tend to use very tightly woven fabrics and/or UV-absorbing chemicals applied to the fabric, and they should include an ultraviolet protection factor (UPF) rating that indicates how much of the sun's UV radiation is absorbed (look for a rating of at least thirty). Wear and tear may reduce the garment's sun protection,

so follow the label's care instructions closely. You can also wash chemical sunscreens into your regular clothes by adding a product like SunGuard to a load of laundry.

The Takeaway: Sun Smarts

Use a broad-spectrum sunscreen that shields you from both UVA and UVB rays. Add to your protection by choosing one that also includes vitamins C and E and/ or EGCG.

When you're outdoors, wear a wide-brimmed hat and tightly woven (but loose-fitting) dark clothing, or clothing specifically designed for sun protection. Wash sunscreen into your clothes in the laundry with a product like SunGuard.

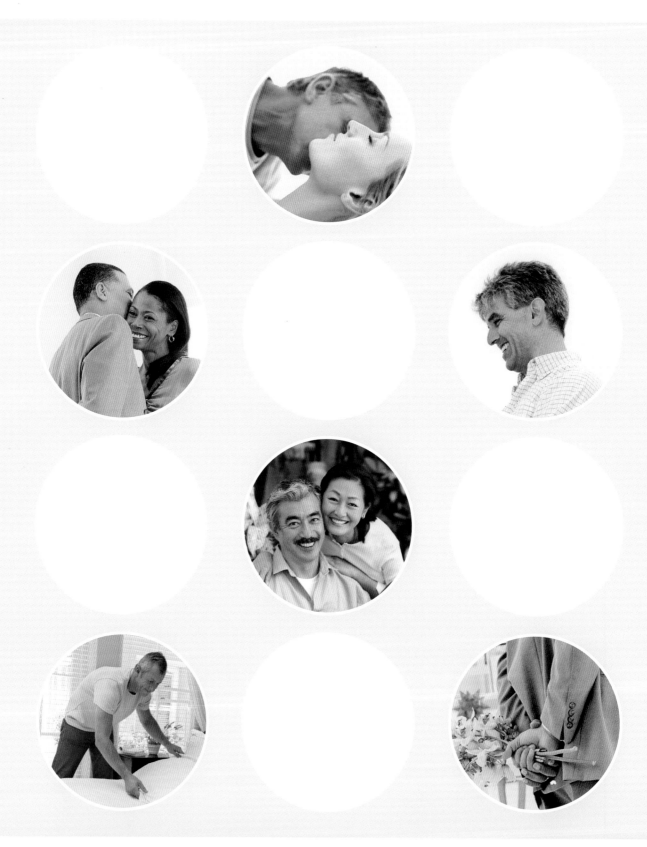

PART VII

Turn Back the Clock on Your Sex Life

12

Address Underlying Health Issues for a Longer Love Life

Need another reason to keep up your healthy habits? People who consider themselves in good health are nearly twice as likely to be interested in sex in middle and older age, report University of Chicago researchers. And respondents to a 2004 AARP survey of older adults said that they believed better health would improve their sex life more than any other factor. Research backs that up: The healthier you are as you get older, the more years of good sex you can have, according to a 2010 study in the *British Medical Journal*. The researchers looked at a group of three thousand adults age fifty-seven to eighty-five and, based on their survey responses, calculated that at age fifty-five, the sexually active life expectancy was 15 years for men and 10.6 years for women. Men in very good or excellent health gained an average of five to seven years of sexually active life beyond that, compared with men in

poorer health. For women in the study, being in very good shape added three to six more years of a superior sex life.

In another study of sexual activity among older adults in the United States, researchers found that men and women who said they had poor health were less likely to be sexually active, and even those who were sexually active reported having more sexual problems. Still, only 38 percent of men and 22 percent of women in the study said they had discussed sex—including the sexual effects of their health conditions—with a doctor since they turned fifty.

Health problems like arthritis or rheumatism, diabetes, high blood pressure, heart disease, and depression can all affect desire and sexual performance. While preventing these conditions in the first place is ideal,

treating them or addressing the problematic symptoms can help you have satisfying sex for years to come.

Treat the Conditions to Lengthen Your Sex Life

Stiff, sore joints or chronic pain can make sexual contact uncomfortable and interfere with intimacy. Try the tips in part IV to keep your joints flexible and reduce pain, and experiment to see if sex is more comfortable for you at different times—in the morning or evening, after exercising, or after a warm bath, for example. Changing positions may also help (for example, try lying on your side, or having the partner with less pain on top). Some pain medications affect sexual function, so talk to your doctor if you think they're causing side effects.

Diabetes, and the obesity that usually accompanies it, can cause erectile dysfunction (ED) in some men. Researchers aren't as sure how diabetes affects women's sexuality, but a 2009 study in the *Journal of Sexual Medicine* found that diabetic women were more likely to have trouble reaching orgasm. In another small study, women with diabetes more frequently reported reduced sexual drive, arousal, vaginal lubrication, orgasm, and overall satisfaction than nondiabetic women—and the longer they'd had diabetes, the worse the sexual problems. Diabetes also increases the risk of vaginal yeast infections, which can make sex uncomfortable. Lifestyle changes (including eating a healthier diet, losing weight, and exercising) and drugs to control blood sugar can help restore sexual function in both men and women.

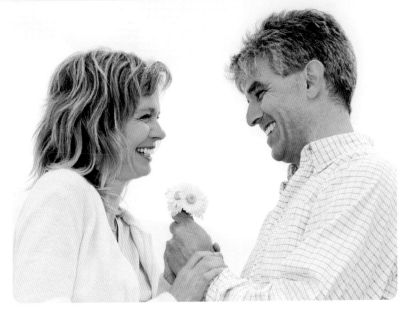

About two-thirds of men with high blood pressure note problems with ED, and hypertension-related ED tends to be worse than in men with normal blood pressure. Women with hypertension are also more than twice as likely to report sexual dysfunction, notes a 2006 study in the *Journal of Hypertension*. Common hypertension drugs such as diuretics and beta-blockers can also have sexual side effects, such as lowered libido, ED, and delayed orgasm in women (▶**73**). Switching drugs or lowering blood pressure through lifestyle changes (▶**52**) can put the sizzle back into your sex life.

Heart disease is linked to ED in men, and they share the same primary risk factors: high LDL ("bad") cholesterol, smoking, hypertension, and diabetes. In fact, men with ED are twice as likely to die from cardiovascular disease, notes a 2010 study in *Circulation*. Changes to blood vessels also reduce blood flow, which can cause both men and women to have trouble with orgasms. Most patients with stable heart conditions can safely be sexually active, and treatment for ED and to improve blood vessel health (such as controlling hypertension and cholesterol) can make sex more enjoyable.

Up to half of people with untreated depression report some type of sexual dysfunction. Unfortunately, several common drugs to treat it bring unwelcome sexual side effects (▶**73**). To restore the luster to your love life, try natural mood boosters such as exercise

and social interaction to help raise your spirits—they may even allow you to lower your dose of medication. And ask your doctor if switching medications might help.

The Takeaway: Health and Sex

Prevent or treat health problems such as arthritis, diabetes, high blood pressure, heart disease, and depression to add years to your sex life.

Try natural treatments such as exercise and social interaction to control underlying conditions; medication side effects often include reduced desire or other sexual problems.

73

Check Medication Side Effects That Age You Sexually

A natural decline in hormone levels may make a difference in sexual response by midlife for both men and women. Complicating matters, health problems such as heart disease, atherosclerosis, high blood pressure, diabetes, and depression can also cause difficulties with arousal and orgasm, vaginal dryness, and erectile dysfunction (▶72).

But it pays to look into another surprising factor behind a sluggish sex drive: Many medications prescribed to treat the very conditions causing sexual complications can actually lower libido, weaken arousal, and make erectile dysfunction (ED) worse. Drugs for high blood pressure and depression are the worst culprits, but they're certainly not the only ones to blame. The drugs cause sexual problems in a variety of ways. And if you take more than one of these medications, the combination of effects can really take a toll in the bedroom.

Beware of Hypertension Drugs That Harm Your Sex Life

The authors of a study in *Current Hypertension Reports* noted that some classes of blood pressure drugs, such as diuretics and beta-blockers, have a greater impact on sexual function than others. While people react quite differently to various hypertension medicines, sometimes even within the same class, these two commonly prescribed classes seem to cause the most problems. Diuretics dilate blood vessels and reduce fluid levels in the body, and beta-blockers act on your nervous system to counter stress-related spikes in blood pressure. Both have been shown to lower libido, contribute to ED in men, and delay orgasm in women. For instance, a 2009 study in the *Journal of Internal Medicine* noted that common side effects of beta-blockers include fatigue,

depression, and sexual dysfunction—all of which can have serious consequences for your love life. And in an earlier study in the *Archives of Internal Medicine*, researchers noted that "Patients taking diuretics reported significantly greater sexual dysfunction than control subjects, including decreased libido, difficulty in gaining and maintaining an erection, and difficulty with ejaculation." Other classes of blood pressure drugs may pose less risk. In fact, research shows that angiotensin II receptor blockers, or ARBs, may actually improve sexual function in men.

Some Antidepressants Interfere with Arousal

A slew of studies show that selective serotonin reuptake inhibitor (SSRI) antidepressants such as Prozac, Paxil, and Zoloft are notorious for dampening desire, partly because of the way they affect neurotransmitters and other hormones and enzymes that impact your central nervous system. In fact, a study in the *Annals of Pharmacotherapy* noted that up to 60 percent of SSRI users experience some kind of sexual repercussions, from delayed or nonexistent orgasm to limited libido and ED. And a 2009 review in the *Journal of Clinical Psychopharmacology* reported that sexual side effects are "one of the predominant reasons" people stop taking the drugs. Monoamine oxidase inhibitor (MAOI) antidepressants and tricyclic antidepressants are less frequently prescribed to treat depression these days, but studies show they may also trigger sexual side effects. Drugs like bupropion (Wellbutrin), which helps balance levels of the neurotransmitters dopamine and norepinephrine, and duloxetine (Cymbalta), which targets both serotonin and norepinephrine, may be less likely to cause problems.

Other Drugs Can Also Dampen Desire

In addition to these main offenders, statins have been linked to ED in men, and prescription or over-the-counter decongestants and antihistamines that dry up your runny nose can also increase vaginal dryness. Drugs for treating heart disease, acid reflux, prostate problems, pain, anxiety, and insomnia (specifically benzodiazepines) often boast unwelcome sexual side effects as well, and your doctor may not think to mention those drawbacks when prescribing.

If you suspect side effects are interfering with your sex life, before you resign yourself to a less-passionate future or turn to ED drugs such as Viagra and Cialis, ask your doctor about reducing your dose, switching to another medicine, or if there are lifestyle approaches to improve the underlying health condition without drugs. And of course, never stop taking a medication without checking first with your doctor.

The Takeaway: Sexual Side Effects

Diuretics and beta-blockers prescribed for hypertension can cause fatigue, lowered libido, and sexual dysfunction.

SSRI antidepressants such as Prozac, Paxil, and Zoloft frequently cause sexual side effects significant enough to cause people to discontinue taking them.

Over-the-counter decongestants and antihistamines can increase vaginal dryness.

14 Increase Your Sexual Confidence As You Age

As you get older, shifts in your appearance may make you more self-conscious and less willing to reveal yourself physically to your partner. That can hamper your love life, and, not surprisingly, a 2009 *Prevention* magazine survey indicates that body embarrassment is more of an issue for women as they age. That's not to say men don't get self-conscious about their appearance, but they're less likely to let it limit their libidos. Self-confidence is always sexy, no matter your age, and research shows that better body image can boost sex drive, even if you've noticed it dwindling over the years. For example, a 2009 study in the *Archives of Sexual Behavior* found that women who felt better about their bodies reported greater sexual desire. Feelings about sexual attractiveness and concern about weight—two factors the researchers used to measure body

confidence—were most significantly related to desire, possibly because those aspects are most on display during sexual intimacy. So cultivating a positive body image can pay off in the bedroom.

A 2009 study in the *Journal of Sex Research* found that for both men and women, positive sexual self-esteem was critical for keeping up their sexual desire in later life. In addition, maintaining self-confidence in all areas of life as you get older can ensure a more passionate love life for years to come. For example, a 2006 study showed that women over the age of sixty-five who had high general self-esteem and stable partners had more sexual experiences than those who had neither. Ready to liven up your love life? Try these tips to increase your own or your partner's self-confidence.

List Your Ageless, Lust-Worthy Qualities

Both bodies and life circumstances change over time, and what you used to take pride in (a flat stomach, work accomplishments) may no longer apply or have lost some luster. But rather than wishing you were twenty-five again, celebrate yourself as you are now to help restore your self-confidence and even refresh your romantic life. To start, make a list of ten things you like about yourself; compile it in your head or write it down to refer to when you need a lift. Try to include both physical attributes (strong shoulders, sparkling eyes) and character traits (generous, quick to laugh) that make you feel attractive. You and your partner can create lists for each other as well—simply knowing that your partner finds you desirable can send your self-esteem soaring, and you might be surprised at what he or she finds alluring about you!

Exercise Makes You Feel Sexy No Matter Your Age

Of course, exercise can help you regain a youthful figure (▸20) and increase sexy muscle definition (▸21), which may help you feel better about revealing your body in the bedroom. But exercise is also one of the best ways to increase your self-confidence regardless of your age or shape. A 2008 study in the *Journal of Physiology and Pharmacology* found that middle-aged, obese women who exercised at least twice a week for two months rated their appearance better than their nonexercising peers did, no matter their weight. Exercise also increases blood flow to body parts involved in arousal (▸76) and triggers the release of mood-boosting endorphins; both may spike your self-confidence and make you more willing to pursue a passionate encounter with your partner.

Do Something You're Good At to Feel Sexually Attractive

Because it tends to strongly influence your sense of identity, self-esteem, and self-worth in all areas of life—including your sexuality—it's worth making sure you enjoy your occupation or avocation, note researchers in a 2009 study in the *Journal of Women's Health & Gender-Based Medicine.* That may mean seeking extra responsibility at work, volunteering, renewing friendships, or making more

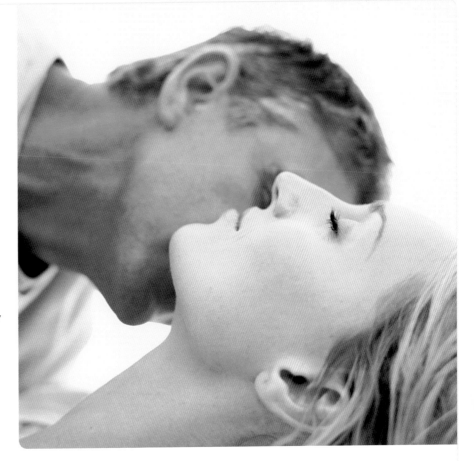

time for a hobby. Any activity that allows you to excel will reward you with greater self-confidence, whether or not you receive recognition for your efforts. That renewed sense of self-worth can spill over into the bedroom. Likewise, seeing your partner shine can be a turn-on.

The Takeaway: Sexy Confidence

Make a list of ten things you like about yourself, including physical attributes and character traits.

Exercise to release endorphins, feel better about yourself, and boost blood flow to sexual body parts.

Do work you enjoy and pursue your hobbies; your success in these endeavors will lead to greater self-esteem.

75

Practice Mindfulness to Renew Romance in Midlife

Although it can enhance your love life at any age, learning to be present in the moment is particularly important for intimacy as you get older. For one thing, it can help stave off bedroom boredom, especially if you've been with your partner for a long time. Tuning in to the physical sensations and emotional aspects of sex can renew your feelings of closeness and make sex more enjoyable. For example, a group of women who received mindfulness training reported that it significantly increased their desire and reduced their sexual distress, while helping them get aroused more easily, according to a 2008 study in the *Journal of Sexual Medicine*.

Additionally, mindfulness practices don't involve reaching a target, and applying that non-goal-oriented approach to sex can take pressure off and even help you redefine what makes a satisfying sexual

experience. Evidence indicates that as people get older, they're not able to climax as easily as they used to. But if orgasm doesn't always have to be the destination, you're free to enjoy the ride, so to speak. Relieving the pressure of performance may be one reason why yoga can help treat premature ejaculation in men, and why mindfulness practices improve several aspects of sexual response and reduce sexual distress in women with desire and arousal disorders (which are more common the older you get), suggests a 2008 review of studies.

Master Your Mind for Better Sex for Years to Come

While you probably didn't need a study to tell you this, research demonstrates that distraction decreases sexual response. Meditation and other mindfulness practices help you learn how to counter that distraction so you can keep your

mind from going in a million different places and enjoy the present, which is especially helpful in the face of flagging desire. Focusing your attention can increase sexual arousal, notes a 2009 study in the *Journal of Sexual Research*. Therefore, since preliminary evidence suggests mindfulness techniques may boost your ability to focus over time, these techniques may ultimately enhance sexual response and satisfaction, the researchers concluded. They may also increase your body confidence: A 2009 study in the journal *Body Image* found that several aspects of mindfulness, such as being able to observe and describe internal and external experiences, significantly affected sexual body esteem in women.

Learning to be more mindful doesn't take a lot of effort—it simply involves slowing down and paying closer attention to your surroundings. If setting aside fifteen minutes to practice mindfulness as part of meditation appeals to you, go for it. But you can also reap the benefits by sneaking in a few mindful moments here and there. You may find it easier to begin in a nonsexual setting. Use all your senses to observe the world around you, such as the smell of a candle or the sound of a clock ticking. When it's comfortable, try applying that to sex—think about what kissing tastes like, the feel of your skin on the sheets, the smell of your partner's hair. Noticing these details can help you reclaim your desire for and enjoyment of sex. By helping you appreciate little things about your partner, it may even restore a spark if your love life has settled into routine.

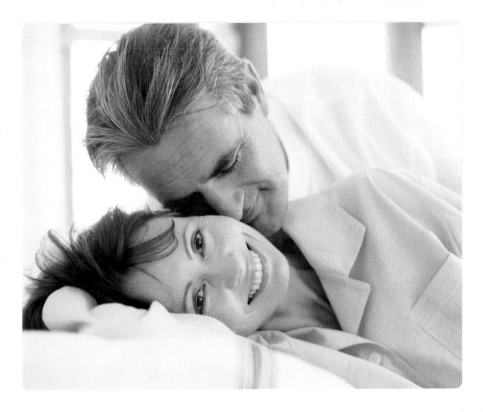

Stretch Regularly to Get More out of Sex

Yoga provides the dual benefits of exercise (▶76) and mindfulness because many of the poses involve balance and focusing on your breath. Maintaining your balance demands concentration—just try standing on one leg while you're mentally rehashing your to-do list—and while breathing generally comes pretty naturally, taking deep breaths or breathing in a pattern requires some thought. A 2009 study in the *Journal of Sexual Medicine* found that after practicing yoga for twelve weeks, women rated several aspects of sexual function (desire, arousal, lubrication, orgasm, satisfaction, and pain) better

than at the start of the study. Notably, women over age forty-five reported more improvement than the younger volunteers did.

While yoga has a long tradition of benefiting sexuality, regularly performing any kind of stretching and balance exercises will offer similar effects as long as you treat them as an opportunity to focus your attention. You can also stretch with your partner, allowing you to connect with each other in a different, but still physical, way.

The Takeaway: Mindful Sexuality

Practice mindfulness daily by staying present in the moment, rather than allowing your mind to race or wander.

Be aware of the sensations of physical intimacy: the sight of your partner's body, the smell of his hair, the touch of skin upon skin.

Stretch or practice yoga to loosen your body while focusing your mind.

76

Exercise to Reverse Age-Related Sexual Problems

Want good sex for a lifetime? Get off the couch! Exercise gives you energy (▶86), relieves stress, triggers the release of mood-boosting endorphins, helps you reconnect with your body, improves health conditions that can interfere with sex (▶72), and can help you lose weight and feel more confident. It also increases blood flow, muscle tone, and agility, all of which decline with age but are critical for arousal and performance, balance, and being able to hold sexual positions comfortably.

While people tend to report more sexual complaints as they get older, such as lowered libido or erectile dysfunction (ED), exercise seems to counteract those problems. For example, a 2010 study in the *Journal of Women's Health* noted that the hormonal shifts of menopause can decrease sexual desire in women, but those who reported having better health and exercising regularly had

significantly more desire than their peers. Similarly, women ages forty-one to sixty-eight said that they participated in sexual activities more frequently and enjoyed sex more if they were physically active, according to a 2009 University of Pittsburgh School of Medicine study. For men, a 2010 review of studies noted that exercise has been shown to improve sexual response and even reverse ED, as well as benefit overall cardiovascular health.

Start with Aerobic Exercise for Better Sex As You Age

Any kind of activity that gets your heart pumping will boost blood flow to all parts of your body, including your genitals, which can increase arousal and lead to better sexual performance. In fact, improvement in blood vessel health is one reason why exercise is so effective in treating ED, suggests a

2010 review of studies in the *Journal of Sexual Medicine*. Exercise also activates the sympathetic nervous system, which is involved in the early stages of sexual arousal and may enhance sexual response, according to a review of studies by researchers at the University of Texas at Austin.

Try to do at least thirty minutes of exercise a day on most days of the week. Breaking it up into ten-minute chunks will still benefit your body if that's the only way you can squeeze it in, but try to make a few of your sessions longer to increase your endurance and keep your blood vessels young and healthy.

Step Up Your Strength Training for More Confident Lovemaking

Resistance exercise, whether you use weights, elastic bands, or your own body weight, increases muscle tone and strength—and that can enhance your sexual response and ability. It can also help you feel more confident with your clothes off: University of Houston researchers found that as little as six weeks of strength training significantly improved how men and women rated their appearance and body satisfaction. To build muscle, do strength exercises twice a week on nonconsecutive days for thirty minutes or more. Be sure to work all your major muscle groups: chest, upper back, shoulders, biceps, triceps, quadriceps (quads), hamstrings and glutes, calves, and abdominal muscles.

In addition to traditional strength moves, you may have heard that exercises targeting your pelvic floor muscles, called Kegels, can increase pleasure and sexual satisfaction in women, since pregnancy and childbirth can weaken those muscles. But aging also affects pelvic floor muscles—in both men and women. That means Kegels can actually benefit men as well. Kegels increase blood flow and muscle tone to pelvic floor muscles, which improve vaginal intercourse. In men, they can help fight ED, which occurs more frequently as you get older: In a 2005 study of men who did Kegels every day for three months, 75 percent regained or improved sexual function. And for both men and women, they can help prevent urinary incontinence down the road. To do a Kegel, tighten your pelvic muscles as if you were stopping the flow of urine. For sexual benefits, do ten Kegels several

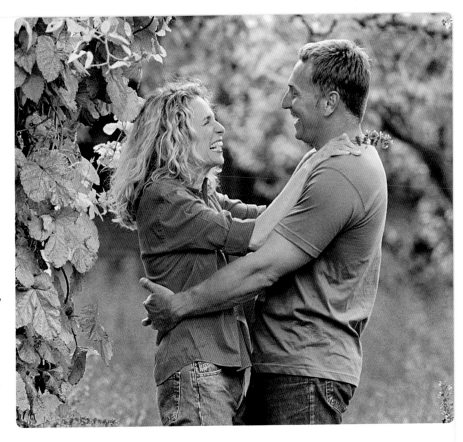

times a day for eight to twelve weeks. You can do them anywhere (in the car, while watching TV) or incorporate them into standard moves like crunches. Remember, just like any other strength exercise, you have to keep it up to maintain the benefits!

The Takeaway: Exercise for Sex

Exercise increases blood flow, muscle tone, and sexual agility, while releasing feel-good hormones and helping you lose weight.

Get your heart pumping with aerobic exercise to counteract low libido and erectile dysfunction.

Do Kegels and consistent strength training to restore desire and improve sexual function.

77

Lift Weights to Boost Fading Testosterone

With age, levels of the sex hormone testosterone decrease in both men and women, which researchers suspect is one reason why older adults tend to have a lower sex drive and report more sexual problems. A 2010 study in the journal *American Family Physician* notes that low testosterone levels are likely responsible for lowered libido and erectile dysfunction (ED) in some men. In a 2007 study, Italian researchers reviewed population research and found that diminished levels of testosterone have a negative impact on desire and sexual responsiveness for midlife and older women as well. (Women produce testosterone in their ovaries, and levels decline—along with estrogen—during menopause.) On the other hand, menopausal women with higher testosterone levels reported significantly greater sexual desire, according to a 2010 study in the *Journal of Women's Health*.

Some studies have investigated whether supplementing with testosterone can restore sexual function and libido in men, with moderately positive results. Other research shows that when women with surgically induced menopause (whose levels of testosterone drop dramatically after removal of their ovaries) are treated with testosterone, they experience significant increases in sexual satisfaction and activity. However, more studies need to be done on the long-term safety of testosterone therapy in men and women, especially since early evidence suggests there's an increased risk of prostate cancer for men. Supplemental testosterone is not recommended for men with marginally low testosterone levels unless they show clinical symptoms of a deficiency. Currently, women in the United States can only get testosterone preparations by having a doctor prescribe them

off-label (that is, not for their intended, Food and Drug Administration [FDA]–approved, purpose).

But there are natural ways to increase testosterone, including exercise. Interestingly, waning testosterone levels seem to be partly responsible for reduced muscle strength in older adults. Exercise can reverse that trend. Obesity is also associated with reduced testosterone levels, and further compounding the problem, declining testosterone signals your body to store more fat around your middle. That suggests that another one of exercise's benefits on testosterone may have to do with helping you stay at a healthy weight. Strength training, in particular, can stimulate the release of testosterone—and thereby restore dwindling desire as you get older.

Make Strength Training a Lifelong Habit

If you needed more motivation to make resistance exercises a nonnegotiable part of your routine, here it is: The most significant testosterone increases seem to occur in people who strength train consistently. Both men and women who strength trained regularly increased their testosterone levels after a single weight-lifting session, found a 2009 study by University of Connecticut researchers. A similar pair of studies in the *Canadian Journal of Applied Physiology* and the *Journal of Sports Medicine and Physical Fitness* found that resistance exercises increased testosterone levels in men, and the effect was greater in those who had lifted weights on a regular basis over the previous several years.

Studies have tested several different workout variations for their effects on hormone levels, and some evidence shows that working large muscle groups at a moderate to high intensity with short periods of rest tends to produce the highest increase in testosterone. Incorporate these guidelines into twenty to thirty minutes of strength training two or three times a week, working all your major muscle groups, and giving your muscles a day to rest in between sessions.

To continue increasing your testosterone levels, you need to keep pushing yourself, suggests a 2008 study in the *Journal of Strength and Conditioning Research*. Your muscles adapt to a routine within about four weeks, so it's important to switch up your moves, the intensity (the amount of weight you use), or the number of repetitions you do to continue challenging yourself and seeing strength (and testosterone!) gains. Fitness magazines and exercise videos are a great source for new ideas and routines.

Don't feel like lifting weights today? You can take a day off every now and then: In addition to exercise, cuddling can increase testosterone levels in women, according to a 2007 study in the journal *Hormones and Behavior*.

The Takeaway: Increase Your Testosterone

Diminished levels of testosterone have a negative impact on desire and sexual responsiveness in both men and women.

Strength training stimulates the release of testosterone.

Do twenty to thirty minutes of strength training two or three times a week, working all your major muscle groups, and giving your muscles a day to rest in between sessions.

78

Enlist All Your Senses to Restore Youthful Desire

With the natural decrease in desire many people experience as they get older, you may find it takes a little extra effort to get in the mood and have satisfying sex. Appealing to all your senses pays off in increased interest in sexual activity, easier arousal, better performance, and overall greater enjoyment in lovemaking—all things that often decline as you get older. So it's definitely worth the effort, wouldn't you say?

Start by addressing the visual, and that doesn't just mean lingerie. Good grooming is important, but you should also clear visual clutter from your bedroom to reduce distraction, and make your bed with your nicest linens. Brush your teeth or pop a mint to make kissing more fun. And put on some mood music, whether you prefer Frank Sinatra, Barry White, neo-punk, or classic rock.

These things may seem minor, but they all send romantic cues to your brain that help set the stage for intimacy.

Get Your Scent On to Lift Your Libido

Scent can be a powerful aphrodisiac, and it may even help counter some of the most common sexual complaints older adults report, such as erectile dysfunction (ED) and vaginal dryness. For example, lavender, reported to soothe stress, may have other sexual benefits as well. Aromatherapy treatment with lavender essential oil (four drops of essential oil diluted with 20 ml of hot water and inhaled for thirty minutes) noticeably reduced cortisol levels and improved blood flow in male volunteers in a 2008 study in the *International Journal of Cardiology*. Better blood flow is linked to superior sexual performance for both men and

women. A warm foot bath with lavender essential oil increases blood flow and the activity of the parasympathetic nervous system, according to a study in the journal *Complementary Therapies in Medicine*. Besides helping you feel more relaxed, the parasympathetic nerves affect men's ability to have and maintain an erection, and in women increase lubrication and enhance the pleasure of sexual stimulation. Another small study confirmed that lavender aromatherapy acts on the autonomic nervous system (which includes the parasympathetic nerves) to simultaneously induce relaxation and increase arousal.

Other sexy scents include pumpkin pie, cucumber, and licorice, according to research from the Smell and Taste Treatment and Research Foundation in Chicago. In men, an odd-sounding combination of lavender and pumpkin pie increased blood flow to the penis by 40 percent, making it a viable alternative to erectile dysfunction drugs. Cucumber and licorice were stronger triggers for women, increasing vaginal blood flow by 13 percent, and thereby boosting arousal. How much a specific scent turns you on has a lot to do with personal preference—and even age. For example, in the above study, the researchers noted that older men tended to respond more strongly to vanilla. And overall, food scents tended to outperform expensive perfumes, perhaps because we already have positive associations with them.

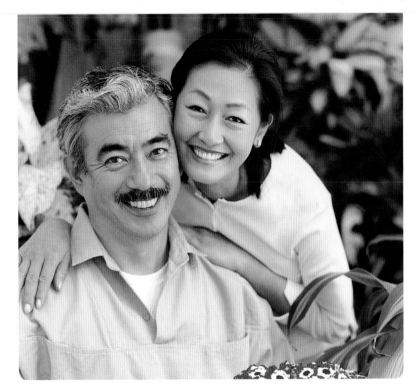

To take advantage of a scent's stimulating qualities, light some candles, use a scented body wash in the shower or bath, or mix essential oils into unscented massage oil for a sensual treat. You can also make your own linen spray by combining 3 ounces (90 ml) of distilled water with about thirty drops of your favorite or a combination of essential oils (add more or less depending on how strong you want the scent, and use light-colored oils to avoid discoloring your linens). Shake well and spray lightly over your sheets.

Explore Touch to Stimulate Your Sex Drive

A hug, holding hands, and a caress on the cheek are all simple ways to show your affection for your partner, and touching, even in ways that aren't explicitly sexual, can increase arousal. Skin-to-skin contact triggers the release of oxytocin, a powerful hormone that enhances feelings of love and desire. That's one reason why foreplay can liven up your lovemaking. As you get older, you may need to set aside extra time for sensual touching, such as massage or using props such as a silk scarf, to allow you and your partner to get in the mood. Extending foreplay can help increase lubrication for older women with vaginal dryness and make for a more passionate encounter for both partners. You can also experiment with water-based lubricants to make sexual touch more pleasurable.

The Takeaway: Powerful Sensuality

Improve visual foreplay with more than lingerie: Clean your bedroom and make your bed with your nicest sheets.

Delight in smells that arouse desire, particularly lavender and pumpkin pie (for men), and cucumber and licorice (for women). Spray your sheets with an essential-oil mixture of thirty drops to 3 ounces (90 ml) of water.

Play music to soothe your mind and stimulate your libido.

Use the power of touch to increase oxytocin and create more arousing foreplay.

79

Dial Back Stress to Rev Up Your Love Life

Too tired or stressed out for sex? While people in all stages of life may find that to be the case now and then, lack of energy and too much tension can exacerbate the sexual problems that older adults commonly face, such as erectile dysfunction (ED) and diminished desire. (About half of midlife and older women and men who reported any sexual activity in the preceding year also reported at least one bothersome sexual problem, according to a 2007 study in the *New England Journal of Medicine*.) But getting enough rest and addressing stress can make a significant difference in those problems, putting the spark back into your sex life today and helping you stay sexually satisfied well into later life.

Fight Fatigue for Better Sex Year after Year

Fatigue depletes your sex drive, and the older you get, the more likely you are to have trouble sleeping thanks to medications, shifting hormones, changing responsibilities, and chronic conditions. On the other hand, being well rested can restore your libido. To get your forty winks, make sure you dedicate enough time for sleep; avoid eating, drinking, or doing anything stimulating (other than sex) right before bed; reduce or eliminate caffeine and alcohol; keep your bedroom dark and quiet; and set a regular sleep schedule (▶19, 32, 63, 84). Ask your doctor if medications or health problems might be interfering with your sleep, and whether switching drugs or reducing the dose, lifestyle changes, or alternative therapies could help treat the underlying condition without the sleep-stealing side effects.

If you're exhausted, it can be hard to convince yourself to work up enough energy or motivation to pursue a passionate moment. But, as with exercise, taking the first few steps often feels so good that you not only end up enjoying the rest of the journey, but you actually have more energy afterward. Try having sex at the times of day when you have the most get-up-and-go, whether that's first thing in the morning or after a workout. See the tips in part VIII for more ideas on how to raise your energy levels enough to fuel an active sex life.

Stop Mid- and Late-Life Stress from Sapping Your Desire

In addition to everyday stresses, older adults face some uniquely challenging situations, such as retirement, illness, caring for aging parents, and other lifestyle adjustments. Piling stress upon stress may lead to sexual difficulties and strain your relationship. A 2008 population study found that for men and women age fifty-seven to eighty-five, stress and anxiety were linked to several sexual problems, including lack of interest, inability to orgasm, pain during sex, lack of pleasure in sex, and worries about performance. Women noted that tension worsened vaginal dryness as well, while men additionally reported trouble achieving and maintaining an erection and climaxing too early.

As you might suspect, one aspect of stress that most frequently resulted in sexual problems was relationship dissatisfaction, noted the authors in the *Journal of Sexual Medicine*. On the other hand, being happy with your relationship is associated with higher sexual pleasure, increased ability to orgasm for women, and greater sexual interest for men. If you have unresolved relationship problems, consider seeing a therapist to help you work through your issues and restore emotional intimacy.

By age sixty-five, between 15 and 25 percent of men experience impotence, or ED, at least one out of every four times they have sex. In something of a self-perpetuating cycle, the pressure to perform sexually can drain sex drive and actually trigger ED in men. And a 2008 study by German researchers found that men with ED who worry about their sexual performance reported less sexual satisfaction overall. Interestingly, while ED itself can lower desire and

make it difficult to have an orgasm, it seems that stress about performance is even more of a factor. Talk to your doctor about treating health conditions, lifestyle changes, medications, and other strategies that can improve ED.

Finally, don't drink to reduce your stress. While a little alcohol may remove some inhibitions, too much can numb your sex drive, cause erection problems in men, and delay orgasm in women.

The Takeaway: Less Stress, Better Sex

Dedicate enough time for sleep and avoid eating, drinking, or doing anything stimulating (other than sex) right before bed.

See a therapist if you are overwhelmed by stressors common to older people: retirement, caring for aged parents, illness, and so on, or if you have unresolved relationship tension.

Don't drink to relieve stress; alcohol can numb your sex drive.

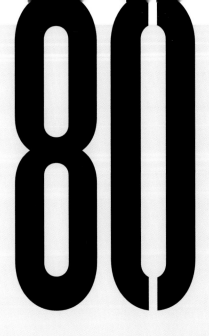

Invest in Nonsexual Intimacy to Extend Your Sex Life

"Age does not protect you from love. But love, to some extent, protects you from age," said actress Jeanne Moreau. Put another way, if you want to stay young, you need to nurture the love in your life. All relationships have ups and downs, and long-term relationships have accumulated years of them. Unresolved or long-simmering problems can make you feel more distant from your partner and dampen desire over time. Lack of intimacy makes it all too easy to fall into a routine (and can make you less willing to break out of one). But emotional closeness is a critical component of a satisfying sex life, especially for women—without it, you may feel like you're just going through the motions. Spending more nonsexual intimate time together can rebuild trust, improve communication, and allow you to express affection for your partner in new ways, helping you navigate the sometimes-rocky road of long-term relationships.

Men and women typically report lower sexual desire as they get older. Some evidence indicates that more than 50 percent of women experience low libido after menopause, and half of men over age fifty report at least occasional erection problems, which can lead to more subdued sexual responsiveness. For older adults experiencing a natural decline in desire, restoring emotional closeness may naturally shift your sex drive out of neutral.

Pursue Emotional Closeness to Preserve Desire

One of the great joys of new relationships is exploration—learning about your partner's likes and dislikes, hopes, and dreams for the future. Those kinds of conversations build intimacy, whether you have them two months or twenty years into your relationship. Older couples may find it takes some effort to continue pursuing their partners long-term, but reaching out can promote a return to the heady days of your early relationship, restoring that sexual spark that used to come so easily. If all you and your partner have talked about for years is the logistical stuff of everyday life, you might be surprised at how you've each changed. So ask again about goals, dreams, and other emotionally invested topics. And then listen, really listen, to the answers. Even in a long-lasting relationship, it can feel risky to share deeply personal thoughts, so this kind of open communication builds trust.

You've probably heard the advice to make regular dates with your mate. Setting aside time for just the two of you cultivates closeness, but it also communicates that your partner is a priority, that you don't take him or her for granted even if you've been together forever, and that your relationship is important enough to nurture. Find other ways to make your partner feel desirable, whether that's complimenting a new piece of clothing, expressing appreciation for a thoughtful action, or suggesting you take a long walk together. And don't expect your mate to read your mind—if you'd like your partner to do something specific to enhance your emotional intimacy, talk about it openly.

If unresolved conflicts make you feel distant, consider couples therapy. A skilled counselor can help you navigate sources of tension and learn how to fight fair. Your therapist may also have suggestions for how to meet each other's emotional needs.

Enjoy Nonsexual Touch to Restore Passion

With skin-on-skin contact, you experience a rush of the "love hormone" oxytocin. If you touch your partner regularly, those levels can stay elevated and reignite fading sexual desire in later life. A 2008 study in the journal *Psychosomatic Medicine* found that couples assigned to a "warm touch" intervention (including hugging, massage, and other physical displays of affection) for four weeks had higher levels of oxytocin throughout the study. Another study discovered that the oxytocin surge was even higher in couples who felt like they had more support from their partner, which underscores the importance of emotional intimacy to physical responsiveness.

That boost of oxytocin can encourage romance, but the touch itself shouldn't always be sexual or come with the expectation that it will lead to sex. Snuggle while you watch TV, give your partner a neck rub after a long day, hold hands when you walk, offer a goodbye kiss as you head out of the house, and welcome your partner home with a hug. Find ways to connect outside the bedroom, and you'll ultimately enjoy more quality time between the sheets.

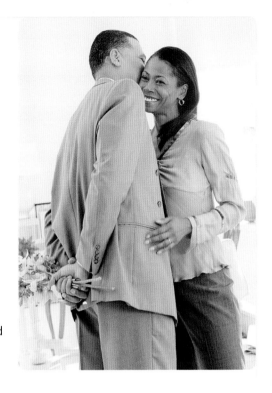

The Takeaway: Nonsexual Intimacy

Talk to your partner about each other's hopes and dreams for the future.

Make your relationship a priority by going on regular dates.

Express your love and appreciation in a variety of ways—compliment your partner or say thank you for doing mundane chores, look for ways to serve, hold hands in public, bring home a thoughtful and unexpected gift, or offer to participate in your partner's favorite hobby.

Use the power of skin-on-skin touch to release oxytocin, "the love hormone."

81

Discuss Shifting Needs and Desires to Increase Satisfaction As You Get Older

Aging affects your sex life in physical and emotional ways. But just because things don't work like they did when you were in your twenties doesn't mean you can't have passionate, fulfilling sex. For example, in a group of women between the ages of forty-five and eighty, an average of 43 percent reported having at least moderate sexual desire, and half of the sexually active participants described their overall sexual satisfaction as moderate to high, according to a 2009 study in the *Journal of the American Geriatrics Society*. Around 60 to 70 percent of men in that age range also reported moderate to high sexual desire in a 2005 study in the *Journal of Sex Research*.

While those numbers tend to go down as you get older, staying in good overall health can help you maintain an active, healthy sex life for longer (▶72). You may need to redefine what makes for a satisfying sexual experience over time, however. Understanding natural changes in desire, arousal, and satisfaction can help you accept them and adapt your lovemaking to ease sexual difficulties and explore new aspects of your sexuality. Talking openly with your partner is also critical, especially so he or she doesn't misinterpret physical changes as a lack of interest.

Learn about Physical Changes As You Age

Talk to your doctor about how aging, illnesses, menopause, and medications might affect your sex life. Knowing how your body (and your partner's) works and what is a healthy sexual response can ease anxiety. For example, men's testosterone levels decline with age, which can lead to lower libido, needing more time and stimulation for erection and orgasm, shorter orgasms, and taking longer to achieve another erection after ejaculation. Women might notice more vaginal dryness, lower desire, or that hot flashes are keeping them up at night and leaving them exhausted (and not exactly in the mood) during the day. Confide in your partner about whatever changes you're experiencing so you can work together to find ways of being intimate that both of you can enjoy.

You should also know that sexual activity falls into the use-it-or-lose-it category: Having sex regularly makes it easier and more enjoyable to continue having sex as you get older. As women go through menopause and their estrogen levels drop, the vaginal walls become thinner and less elastic. However, sexual activity that involves penetration can slow or even reverse this process. For men, going for a long time without an erection can lower blood flow to the penis and actually reduce the muscle cells' ability to expand when blood flow does increase, making it harder to achieve and maintain an erection. But having sex regularly boosts circulation to the genitals, increasing both pleasure and sexual function.

Talk about Concerns and Wants for Lifelong Satisfaction

Good communication is essential for all aspects of a healthy relationship, including sex. If discussing physical intimacy with your partner face to face is too uncomfortable, try writing down your thoughts or reading a book about sexuality together and underlining passages that appeal to you. Or seek out a professional counselor who can help you understand what's normal and suggest nonthreatening and encouraging ways to share your feelings about sex with your partner.

It's worth facing a little embarrassment to avoid staying frustrated, unhappy, or depressed about age-related changes, which will only hurt your relationship, and your sex life, more in the long run. Ultimately, being honest can bring you closer to your partner and help you both enjoy sex and intimacy more.

As you discuss the physical and emotional changes you're going through, describe what you enjoy about sex. You might be surprised to learn that your partner doesn't necessarily want to have intercourse all the time, but enjoys sensual touching, kissing, and other intimate sexual contact that meets emotional and physical needs. Maybe your partner's sex drive hasn't dipped at all as you've gotten older. Or perhaps you feel that sex has become too predictable, and you'd like to try new techniques or positions (▶ 82). Find compromises that incorporate pleasurable activities for both of you.

The Takeaway: Talk Openly for Better Sex

Honesty sparks intimacy: Discuss your physical and emotional changes with your partner.

Older men might need more time and stimulation for erection and orgasm; older women might experience vaginal dryness, lower desire, and hot flashes at night that disrupt sleep and leave them wiped out.

Use it or lose it! Intercourse can slow the thinning of the vaginal walls, and men who go without an erection for an extended period of time may find it harder to achieve one.

82

Try New Techniques to Refresh a Stale Sex Life or Adapt to Physical Changes

Keeping your romantic life fresh and fun is one way to maintain sexual desire and increase satisfaction as you get older, especially if you've been with your partner for years. "Monotony in sexual relationships, such as predictability of sexual activities and over-familiarity with the partner, may contribute to a loss in sexual desire," notes a 2005 study about sexuality in older adults in the *Journal of Sex Research*. Boredom undermines closeness, which can make you feel less satisfied with your relationship. However, if partners can inject excitement into their relationship from other sources, such as participating in new and challenging activities together, "this shared experience can reignite relationship passion by associating the excitement with the relationship," write the authors of a 2009 study in the journal *Psychological Science*. And

couples who have been together a long time may actually have an advantage over younger paramours in one way: Brain scans indicate that long-term love lights up areas where the "bonding" hormone oxytocin is active.

Experimenting in the bedroom can also help you adapt your physical intimacy to overcome any new sexual limitations you may experience as you get older, such as erectile dysfunction or problems caused by health conditions (▶72). Being willing to try new things helps demonstrate to your partner that you believe sex is—and should continue to be—an important part of your relationship regardless of the physical changes that come with aging.

Break Out of a Rut to Reignite Desire

Novelty boosts the brain chemical

dopamine, according to University College London researchers. Dopamine is linked to the brain's reward center and helps fuel sex drive, and studies show that all kinds of new experiences, images, people, and thoughts can trigger its release. Trying something different with your partner can stimulate the "excitement" receptors in your brain and send dopamine flooding into your system. Because we associate that with reward, it can reinforce a positive connection between you and your partner. In fact, a recent study by Stony Brook University researchers found that couples who participated in a new and challenging experience together rated their relationships better and were more attracted to each other after completing the task.

To take advantage of the dopamine surge and its benefits for your relationship, try a new activity—and it doesn't have to be sexual. Anything out of the realm of your normal experience counts, even if it's something you used to do together but have let fall to the wayside in recent years, like going to a bar or visiting a museum. Explore an unfamiliar walking path together, try tandem biking or kayaking, take in a comedy show, learn a new game, enter a race together, participate in a scavenger hunt, or dream up and host an event to raise money for charity. Celebrating milestones and achievements also cultivates closeness and can rekindle a spark.

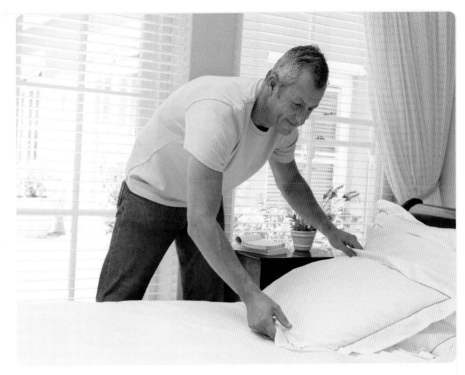

Offset Dwindling Desire with Creativity in the Bedroom

Wearing sexy lingerie, sharing fantasies, role-playing, using sex toys or lubricants, and attempting new positions can all help you break out of a sexual rut. You can also make love in a new location, or even at a different time of day than you're used to. Other suggestions include focusing on using all five of your senses during intimacy to heighten sensual awareness (▶75). Leave steamy love notes for your partner to find later. Break out the whipped cream and chocolate body paint. Take the initiative if you usually let your partner get things started. Explore erotic books or films (or make your own!). Make an extra effort at romantic gestures such as enjoying a picnic together on a lovely day, reading poetry to each other, or writing a song for your partner. You get the idea: Be adventurous and use your imagination

to find something that's new to you and your partner. Even if you end up not enjoying a new position, toy, or technique, simply having experimented with it can inject fresh passion into ho-hum sex. And you may just find an incredibly pleasurable new favorite!

The Takeaway: Incorporate Novelty for Better Sex

Boredom undermines closeness; do something new together to release the "reward" chemical dopamine and reconnect.

Celebrate milestones and achievements to renew a romantic spark.

Get creative in the bedroom with new positions, new times for lovemaking, new scents, or new lingerie.

83

Take Herbs and Supplements to Restore a Sexual Spark

Do an Internet search for supplements to boost sex drive, and you'll get over 1.5 million hits for substances that are largely unproven, usually ineffective, and sometimes even downright dangerous. To help you sort through the hype, here are research-backed supplements that may revive a waning libido, improve erectile dysfunction (ED), and relieve other age-related sexual problems. Always talk to your doctor before taking supplements, natural or not, since many interact with medications or other herbs or may not be safe to take if you have certain health conditions.

ArginMax Increases Sexual Satisfaction

This proprietary supplement combines the amino acid L-arginine and the herbs ginkgo, ginseng, and damiana, plus vitamins and minerals, to increase desire and improve sexual function. Your body

uses L-arginine to make nitric oxide, which relaxes blood vessels and boosts blood flow. Ginkgo has a similar effect. Besides increasing nitric oxide levels, ginseng acts as a mild stimulant and sexual "energizer." Damiana (*Turnera diffusa*) may calm anxiety and is a reputed aphrodisiac, but it hasn't been well studied.

Women going through menopause who took the supplement reported having more sex and being more satisfied with their sexual relationship, as well as having better vaginal lubrication, compared to women taking a placebo, noted a 2006 study in the *Journal of Sex and Marital Therapy*. Additionally, more than half the postmenopausal women in the study reported higher sexual desire. Because it doesn't exert estrogenlike effects, the researchers suggested ArginMax might make a

good alternative to hormone therapy for menopause-related sexual concerns. In an earlier study, nearly 75 percent of people taking ArginMax said they were more satisfied with their sex life, compared with 37 percent of the placebo group. The women also noted higher sexual desire, less vaginal dryness, more frequent intercourse and orgasm, and better clitoral sensation. In a small study investigating ArginMax in men, almost all the volunteers said they were better able to maintain an erection during intercourse, and 75 percent were more satisfied with their sex life.

Men's and women's formulations are available; follow package directions for dosing. Allow four weeks to notice a difference. The supplement seems to be safe—no studies have reported significant side effects.

Give Ginkgo and Ginseng a Try to Improve Arousal

Although they're components of ArginMax, you can take these herbs separately. Ginkgo biloba facilitates blood flow and relaxes smooth muscle tissue while enhancing the effects of nitric oxide, helping men achieve and maintain an erection. In a 2008 *Archives of Sexual Behavior* study, women taking ginkgo for eight weeks along with sex therapy noted greater sexual desire and contentment compared to placebo. Some evidence suggests it may benefit people experiencing sexual side effects from antidepressants (▸**73**). The usual amount is 120 milligrams daily, in divided doses with food. It's relatively safe, although you shouldn't use it while taking blood thinners.

The active compounds in Asian ginseng (*Panax ginseng*), called ginsenosides, increase nitric oxide and relax blood vessels and expandable tissues in the penis that fill with blood during an erection. Men taking ginseng reported better erectile function and overall satisfaction after eight weeks, researchers noted in the *Asian Journal of Andrology*. Search for standardized extracts and follow package dosing directions; allow six to eight weeks to see an effect. Ginseng is generally considered safe, but it can raise blood pressure and cause irritability and insomnia in some people.

Revive a Waning Libido with Maca

Early evidence indicates that maca (*Lepidium meyenii*), a Peruvian root traditionally used as an aphrodisiac, may improve desire and sexual function. Maca doesn't appear to affect hormone levels, and researchers aren't sure exactly how it works. But a handful of studies suggest maca may liven up your sex life by improving your general sense of well-being. Men with mild ED who took maca for twelve weeks reported better erections and feeling happier with their sex lives than men taking a placebo, according to a 2009 study in *Andrologia*. In a small 2008 study, Massachusetts General Hospital researchers studied maca in patients taking SSRI antidepressants and found that it boosted libido and improved several measures of sexual function. Postmenopausal women taking maca for six weeks reported less anxiety and depression and a nearly 35 percent improvement in sexual problems compared to placebo, noted a 2008 study in *Menopause*.

Maca seems to be well tolerated and have few side effects. Studies used between 1.5 and 3.5 grams, with 3 grams daily considered a high, but safe and effective, dose.

The Takeaway: Sexual Supplements

ArginMax includes L-arginine (your body uses it to make nitric oxide, which relaxes blood vessels and boosts blood flow), along with gingko, ginseng, and vitamins and minerals. Most people who take it report more satisfaction with their sex lives and no side effects.

Gingko and ginseng, taken separately, increase desire and sexual contentment in men and women.

Maca, a Peruvian root, helps restore libido and sexual function, although researchers aren't sure how.

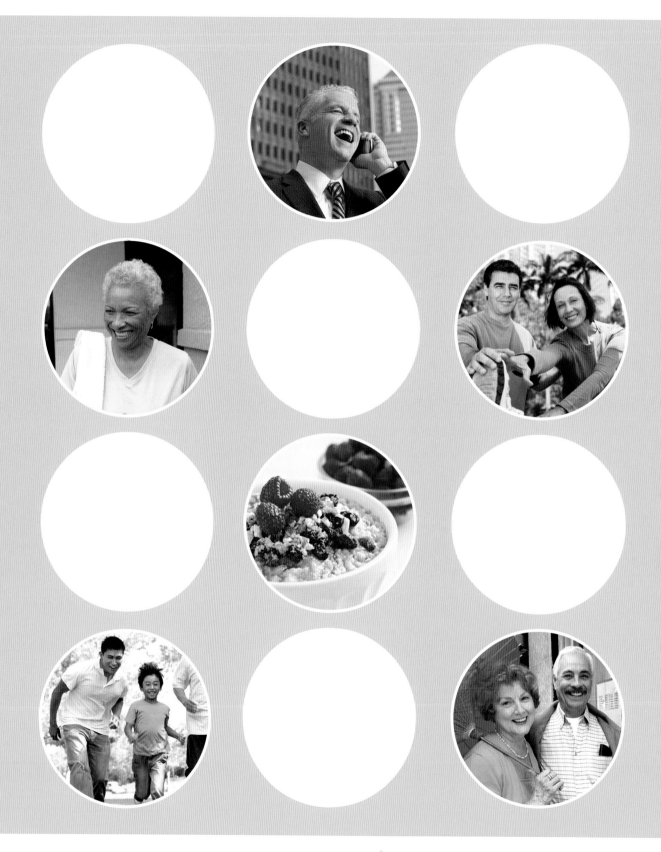

PART VIII

Turn Back the Clock for More Energy

84

Wake Up Refreshed for Lifelong Vitality

While sleep keeps your immune system young (▶63), fends off cognitive decline (▶32), and can even help you combat midlife weight gain (▶19), probably the most obvious benefit to a good night's rest is having enough energy during the day. Once you reach your mid-thirties you may start to notice that you don't have as much energy as you used to. That's partly because of age-related sleep changes, such as shifting circadian rhythms that make you want to go to bed and wake up earlier. The sleep-regulating hormone melatonin also decreases with age, meaning you feel less sleepy at night and may find it harder to doze off. And although experts don't fully understand why, older adults spend less time in deep, energy-restoring sleep, making chronic insomnia a common late-life complaint. Health problems, medications, changing hormones, and stress can also sabotage your slumber—in fact, up to 80 percent of older adults with four or more health problems report poor sleep, according to the National Sleep Foundation. But fatigue is not an inevitable part of aging. The first step in maintaining sky-high energy levels as you get older is to improve the quality (and quantity, if necessary) of your sleep.

Sleep Deeply As You Get Older

Although your risk of sleep problems increases as you get older, you can employ several strategies to ensure satisfying sleep. First, ask your doctor if any of your medications or a health condition might be aggravating insomnia. For example, older adults are more likely to report sleep disorders such as restless legs syndrome or obstructive sleep apnea, according to a 2010 study in the French journal *Psychologie & NeuroPsychiatrie du Vieillissement.* Next, examine your sleep hygiene. To help you nod off, stick to a consistent sleep schedule, avoid stimulating activities before bed, exercise regularly, and use stress-management techniques (▶85) so worry doesn't keep you up.

Once you fall asleep, you want to stay asleep—waking up frequently in the middle of the night pretty much guarantees you'll be wiped out the next day. To minimize interruptions, turn off the TV and radio (or put them on a timer so they don't run all night), keep your bedroom dark, limit late-night liquid intake to reduce trips to the bathroom, and cut back on caffeine and alcohol. If you still have problems sleeping, you may want to try a natural sleep aid like melatonin (▶63). A dose of 0.25 milligrams is safe to take long-term.

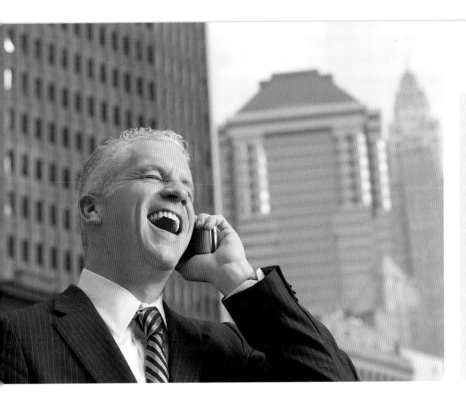

The Takeaway: Rise and Shine

Keep a consistent sleep schedule in a dark bedroom and limit your beverage intake in the evening to avoid nighttime bathroom trips.

If you have trouble sleeping, write down your thoughts in a journal to clear your mind or take a melatonin supplement.

Use light and cold water to rise refreshed and shake off a.m. grogginess. Let the sun stream in through the windows; splash your face with cold water.

Wake Up Well for Daytime Pep

Try these a.m. tactics for all-day energy. Light is one of the most important cues to your circadian clock, according to a 2010 study in the journal *Sleep Medicine Reviews*. Exposing yourself to light first thing in the morning signals to your body that it's time to get up and go, making it easier to bound out of bed. In the summer, you might try sleeping with your curtains open to take advantage of the sunlight streaming in, but when the sun doesn't rise so early, you can use an alarm clock that rouses you from sleep with a light that gradually gets brighter (many have backup measures like beepers to ensure you don't snooze past your set wake-up time).

Another strategy is to get moving as soon as you open your eyes. Instead of lounging in bed, work in some activity right away, whether it's doing a few gentle stretches or dancing along to a favorite song. This gets your blood flowing, loosens your muscles, and gives you a dose of energizing oxygen.

For instant invigoration, give yourself a quick blast of cold water in the shower, splash it on your face, or gargle with it—the sudden temperature change shakes off morning fogginess. If you can't bear the shock of cold water, give yourself an invigorating rubdown with a washcloth or loofah to get your blood flowing (use a body wash or soap with an energizing scent for extra help

waking up). Mint-flavored toothpaste can also give you a subtle boost by acting on a nerve in your brain that helps you feel more energized.

85

Don't Let Stress Slow You Down As You Get Older

Fatigue is a substantial problem for older people, but because it has so many different causes, it's notoriously difficult to treat, noted a 2010 review in the *International Journal of Nursing Studies*. Stress is one factor that can send already-flagging energy levels into a downward spiral. In fact, older adults who are anxious are more likely to show increased fatigue, according to a 2006 study in the *Journals of Gerontology: Psychological Sciences and Social Sciences*. It's no surprise that chronic tension can wear you out—exposure to continuously high levels of stress hormones such as cortisol keep your body in a fight-or-flight response that it just can't maintain long-term, and your energy levels pay the price. Here's how to dial down and put the pep back in your step.

Put an End to Midlife Multitasking

The first order of business is to take care of your health: Eat well, exercise regularly, and get enough sleep. These basics are increasingly important as your natural energy production slows over time. Next, stop trying to do too many things at once. You may think that multitasking helps you be more efficient with your time, and to some extent— like washing the dishes while talking on the phone, or listening to a book on tape during your commute—that can be true. But trying to do more than one task that requires similar levels of attention, like paying bills while talking on the phone, means that neither gets your full concentration. Ultimately, it takes longer to do both because you're constantly breaking focus to switch between them, which can skew your perception of how much you actually have to do, unnecessarily increasing stress and making you feel frazzled.

A 2009 study by Stanford researchers found that people who regularly multitask with different forms of media are less able to filter out irrelevant and distracting information, which takes up extra mental space and worsens their focus. Identify the time-stealers that you frequently try to tack on to other tasks. If that's email or Facebook, for example, set aside specific times to check your inbox and respond (twice a day, once an hour, etc.). That frees you to devote complete attention to a job and do it well so you can cross it off your to-do list and move on.

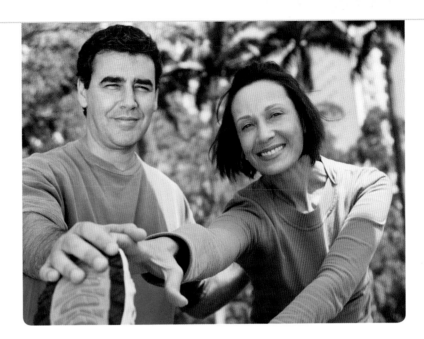

Organizing your time can help calm the anxiety of feeling overwhelmed and lift the sense of overarching dread that so often accompanies it. Instead of letting monster projects—from your company's annual report to your parents' golden wedding anniversary party—hang over your head and drain you, control the chaos by breaking them down into manageable chunks and tackling them one by one. If you don't know where to begin, ask for help prioritizing. Having a greater sense of control can be super stress relieving, allowing you to be more productive in the long run and enjoy the time you have "off" because you know things are progressing on schedule. To help you feel even more in control, be as prepared as you can. For instance, leave enough time for travel, or review your notes before a presentation.

Have Fun Every Day to Live a More Fulfilling Life

Another key to relieving energy-sapping stress as you get older is to make time for things you enjoy. Even if you only have a few minutes, taking a walk outside, reading a chapter in a good book, or calling a friend can refresh your spirits and your energy levels. Inject fun into your life whenever you can for a natural lift: Tell jokes to your coworkers, juggle your groceries as you put them away, listen to music while you do chores. Learn relaxation skills such as deep breathing techniques, guided imagery, and meditation that you can use to unwind whenever you need a moment of peace.

Humor may provide extra stress-squashing benefits, whether you watch a classic comedy or listen to a friend regale you with a sidesplitting anecdote. "Laughter releases excessive physical and psychological energy, and it reduces stress, anxiety, worry, and frustration," note the authors of a study in the *Journal of Gerontological Nursing*. If you find yourself fretting over factors out of your control, seek out witty friends who can divert your attention and help you regain perspective. Besides making difficult situations seem more manageable, the social support busts stress by giving you a safe outlet to share concerns and get feedback—and you'll likely return to the problem with a fresh approach and renewed energy.

The Takeaway: Stress Relievers

Stop trying to do so much at once. Multitasking actually makes you less effective, not more.

Take the time to do the things you enjoy. Spend time outdoors or with a friend, or pair not-so-fun activities (such as chores) with more enjoyable pursuits such as listening to your favorite music.

Laugh more. Watch comedies, go to comedy clubs, and call a witty friend to help you see things in a new light and lighten your stress load.

86

Get Moving to Counteract Age-Related Fatigue

Newton's first law of motion states, in part, that an object at rest tends to stay at rest. That applies to your body too—the longer you're inactive, the more sluggish you'll feel, and the harder it can be to motivate yourself to move—and it's increasingly true as you get older and have less natural get-up-and-go. Older adults who are less active are more likely to report increased fatigue levels, noted Iowa State University researchers in a 2006 study. But the opposite also applies: Increasing your daily activity can send your energy levels skyrocketing.

You may feel wiped out after sitting at a desk all day, but it's easy to confuse being mentally tired with being physically tired. After about forty-five minutes of inactivity, you'll start to feel fatigued. But you can break out of that sedentary stupor just by getting up from your chair. Physical movement is invigorating because it boosts circulation and loosens tight muscles and joints (both of which get worse with age), and it gives your cells a burst of energizing oxygen. Take advantage of those benefits by adding movement throughout your day, especially to break up monotonous tasks or long periods of sitting, or at times when you normally feel like a zombie.

Fight Fatigue with Exercise

Regular low- and moderate-intensity exercise can combat fatigue, according to a 2008 study in the journal *Psychotherapy and Psychosomatics.* Sedentary but otherwise healthy volunteers who complained of constant tiredness reported significantly more energy after exercising for just twenty minutes three times a week for six weeks. What's more, each exerciser reported at least a 49 percent drop in feelings of fatigue. Strength training provides similar benefits, according to a 2009 study in the *Journal of Sports Sciences.* And while you should aim for at least thirty minutes of exercise on most days of the week for good overall health, research shows that even a few minutes of low-intensity movement here and there can stimulate your central nervous system, clearing out mental cobwebs and helping you feel more alert.

Older adults stand and walk less per day than younger people do, according to a 2007 study in the *American Journal of Physiology: Endocrinology and Metabolism.* The researchers suggested that lean, healthy older adults may actually "have a biological drive to be less active than the young." So in addition to your daily workout, as you get older you'll probably have to be intentional in finding ways to add extra activity to your normal routine. Pace while you're on the phone, conduct walking meetings at work, eat at your desk and take a quick walk around the block during your lunch break, or even swap your chair for a stability ball (you have to use your leg and core muscles to keep yourself balanced, and you can also bounce on it from time to time). The more you move, the more lively you'll feel: A 2006 review of population studies in the journal *Sports Medicine* found that higher amounts of physical activity were strongly tied to greater energy and less fatigue. As a bonus, moving more throughout your day can rev up a sluggish midlife metabolism (▶**22**), helping you lose weight and making it even easier to be active. It also ensures you'll be able to stay active well into late life.

Put On a Pedometer to Measure Activity Levels

A pedometer measures how active you really are, and seeing the numbers in black and white can spur you to get moving. Experts recommend getting 10,000 steps (roughly 5 miles, or 8 km) a day for good health, including increased energy. You'll probably find that number is hard to reach without dedicating daily time for a workout, but little bursts of activity quickly add to your total and send your energy soaring. You may also prefer to take an average of your steps over a week so you don't get discouraged by a low-count day. When you do fall short of your goal, use it as an opportunity to brainstorm ways you can overcome that day's roadblocks in the future, such as making a contingency plan for rotten weather or arranging active dates with friends and family.

The Takeaway: Move More to End Fatigue

Get moving to increase energy (and to rev up a sluggish midlife metabolism). Aim for thirty minutes of moderate exercise on most days of the week, or squeeze in ten-minute spurts to fight fatigue.

Wear a pedometer to count your steps; experts recommend that you take 10,000 per day to maintain fitness and stay energized as you age.

87

No More Naps! Eat to Sustain All-Day Energy

Eating energy-stabilizing foods can help revive flagging energy levels as you get older. Your body—especially your brain, which has few energy reserves of its own—needs a steady supply of blood sugar to function at its best, but too much or too little can leave you drained. Filling up on simple carbs or going too long without eating can weaken your body's response to insulin, the hormone that helps you use glucose (sugar) for energy. Besides sapping your strength, over time that insulin resistance can cause high levels of glucose to build up in your blood and set the stage for diabetes, which speeds up aging throughout your body (▶55).

Fortunately, the foods that keep your blood sugar steady also provide nutrients necessary for energy-producing reactions in the body. Rich in vitamins, minerals, and anti-aging antioxidants, this fountain-of-youth fare can restore energy, reduce your risk of age-accelerating diabetes, keep your waistline in check as you get older (see part II), and ensure your body can operate at peak form for years to come.

Fuel Your Body with the Right Foods for Youthful Energy

Snacking is a smart strategy to keep you going when you hit a wall: Most people need to eat every three to four hours to avoid running on empty. But while you may be tempted to reach for a soda or cookies for a quick energy boost, you'll crash just as swiftly. Forcing your body to work extra hard to balance your blood sugar wears you out and leaves you feeling sluggish. Selecting snacks that combine protein, complex carbohydrates, and healthy fats will give you long-lasting energy because your body digests them steadily. Fiber-rich foods also help lower insulin levels and slow the release of sugars into your blood. Recharge with snacks such as whole-grain crackers and cheese, fruit and nuts, plain yogurt with berries and granola, baby carrots and white bean dip, and celery and peanut butter.

Follow the same guidelines for meals as well. Ditch the cornflakes and lift your a.m. fog with a power breakfast of old-fashioned or steel-cut oats, milk, blueberries, pecans, and a sprinkle of blood sugar–lowering cinnamon. Having a large or high-carb lunch can exacerbate the afternoon slump triggered by your circadian rhythms, according to a 2005 study in the journal *Clinics in Sports Medicine*, so downsize your portions and be sure to include protein, fat, and fiber to keep you going strong all afternoon. Make your lunch sandwich on 100 percent whole-wheat bread, add cucumbers and roasted red peppers to your lettuce and tomato, and trade your mayo for fiber- and protein-rich hummus. And for dinner, choose brown rice for your stir-fry, use a small amount of slow-burning lean protein, and double the vegetables (hold the sugary sauce).

Drink Wisely to Boost Your Energy

Even mild dehydration can make you feel tired as you get older, so water should be the first beverage you reach for if you want to perk up. If you aren't hydrated enough, your body fluids can actually thicken slightly, which slows circulation and chemical reactions that produce energy throughout your body, according to a 2007 study in the *Journal of the American College of Nutrition*. How much water you need depends on several factors, including your activity level and climate. Food (especially water-rich fruits and vegetables) can account for about 20 percent of your total fluid intake, according to the Mayo Clinic. In addition to diet, the Institute of Medicine suggests that men consume about thirteen cups (3 L) and women consume about nine cups (2.2 L) of total beverages a day. A good general guideline is that if you feel thirsty or notice your mouth is dry, start sipping.

If you need a caffeine boost, opt for green or black tea instead of coffee. Although tea doesn't contain as much caffeine per cup (only 20 to

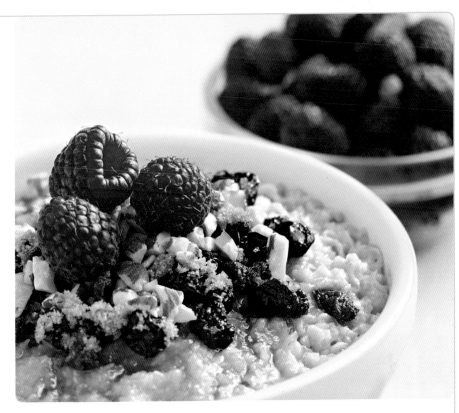

30 milligrams in 8 ounces [240 ml], compared to 100 milligrams in coffee), it has the added benefits of powerful age-fighting antioxidants and stimulants like theophylline and the amino acid L-theanine, which can increase blood circulation, improve oxygen flow, and help you stay alert without feeling jittery. Green and black tea also help insulin regulate your blood sugar more effectively, preventing energy spikes and crashes and reducing your risk of developing type 2 diabetes.

The Takeaway: Eat and Drink for Energy

Eat small snacks every four hours or so to keep your blood sugar steady. Combine protein with complex carbohydrates, such as peanut butter and apples or yogurt and granola.

Drink plenty of water to improve your circulation. For an energy boost, choose green or black tea over coffee for their anti-aging antioxidants.

88

Perk Up with Safe Supplements That Restore Youthful Energy

Yes, caffeine and related stimulants will give you a lift. However, another class of energy-enhancing supplements may revive waning energy levels as you get older without the jittery side effects. Derived from substances already in our bodies or that we get from food, these compounds affect how the body metabolizes the nutrients we eat and translates them into energy, studies show. If you get enough from a healthy, well-balanced diet, popping a pill probably won't help. But if you're deficient because of poor eating habits, strenuous exercise, chronic stress, or regularly taking certain medications (such as acid blockers, anti-inflammatory painkillers, or antibiotics), supplementing might provide some benefit. Keep in mind, however, that lifestyle changes are likely to be far more effective than a supplement. Before taking these or any supplements, talk to your doctor about how they might affect

any medical conditions you have and possible drug interactions.

Boost Flagging Energy with B Vitamins

The B vitamins play an important role in energy production, helping you think clearly and improving sleep quality—and a deficiency makes you feel sluggish. For example, thiamin, or B1, helps nervous system tissue use blood sugar (glucose) to produce energy, and it plays a role in cognitive performance, especially in older adults. And vitamins B6 and B12, among others, are required to synthesize certain energizing neurotransmitters, notes a 2006 study in the *Journal of Nutrition, Health & Aging*.

While most people get enough from food, U.S. Department of Agriculture data indicates that more than one-third of adults age sixty to sixty-nine have

intakes below the recommended daily allowances (RDAs) for vitamin B6 and folate. As you get older, your body is also less able to absorb vitamin B12. Stress depletes the B vitamins as well, and many medications (such as acid blockers, antibiotics, or the antidiabetes drug Metformin) can interfere with absorption. Experts recommend that all adults over fifty take a B-50 complex supplement daily (which provides 50 milligrams of most of the B vitamins, plus 400 micrograms of folic acid) or a multivitamin that provides 100 percent of the RDA for all the B vitamins.

Clear the Cobwebs with CoQ10

Found in the mitochondria, the energy factories of our cells, coenzyme Q10 is critical for producing energy. A powerful antioxidant, CoQ10 also protects you from ever-increasing free-radical attacks on mitochondria as you get older, which interfere with energy production and speed up aging. CoQ10 helped relieve symptoms of chronic fatigue among middle-aged women in a 2005 study in the *Journal of Clinical Psychiatry*. And a 2010 review of studies in the journal *Nutrition* noted that supplementing with CoQ10 can make exercise seem easier by reducing feelings of fatigue during a workout.

With no known side effects, CoQ10 appears quite safe. Although you can get enough from foods, including beef, soybean oil, sardines, mackerel, and peanuts, if you still have low energy (or are at risk for heart problems [▶58]), you might want to supplement to see if it helps. Common medications, such as statins, antidepressants, and antihypertensives, also significantly lower levels of CoQ10. If you're on these medicines, you'll need to supplement to get enough CoQ10. Take 50 to 150 milligrams of the softgel form daily with a meal containing some fat for the best absorption.

Try Tyrosine for Mental Tiredness

Mental fatigue is linked to lower levels of L-tyrosine and other amino acids, according to a 2007 study in the *Journal of Neural Transmission*. You need tyrosine to produce the neurotransmitters dopamine, epinephrine, and norepinephrine. (Tyrosine helps make CoQ10 as well.) But stress, such as sleep deprivation and fatigue, depletes levels of these

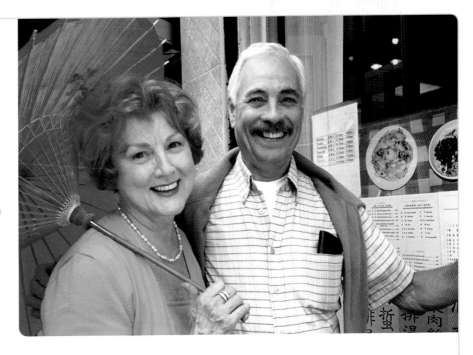

energizing substances, worsening mid- and late-life feelings of fogginess. Supplementing with tyrosine appears to increase mental focus by "reducing the acute effects of stress and fatigue on task performance," suggests a 2009 study in *Alternative Medicine Review*. Other research indicates taking tyrosine can make demanding work seem easier and improve some measures of mental performance. It works quickly to boost energy and alertness (and may even brighten your mood), but tyrosine seems to work best to reinvigorate you during stressful situations.

Take tyrosine on an empty stomach. Experts recommend 500 to 1,000 milligrams daily, and although it appears safe to take indefinitely, you might want to take a monthly break to see if you can do without it. It can cause anxiety and raise blood

pressure in some people, and those with melanoma or phenylketonuria should not take tyrosine.

The Takeaway: Energy-Boosting Supplements

Adults over fifty should take a B-50 complex supplement or a multivitamin with 100 percent of the RDA for B vitamins daily.

Try CoQ10 to relieve physical fatigue and make workouts seem easier.

Tyrosine increases mental energy and alertness, but people with melanoma or phenylketonuria shouldn't take it.

89

Break Out of a Rut to Reignite Your Zest for Life

Feeling weary beyond your years? As you reach mid- or late life, you've had several decades to accumulate ingrained behaviors and ways of thinking. And while familiarity can be comforting, it can also sap your energy. Trying something new or introducing elements of excitement, on the other hand, can restore youthful passion and vigor. If you've fallen into predictable patterns, try these tips to shake things up and feel years younger.

Vary Your Age-Old Routine

Novel activities engage you in life and even help time pass more quickly, rather than monotonously dragging on and draining you, according to a 2010 study in the *American Journal of Occupational Therapy*. Even small changes such as ordering a different drink at the coffee shop or taking a different route to work once or twice a week can help you break out of a life set on automatic pilot. Novelty boosts the "feel-good" brain chemical dopamine, noted a 2006 study in the journal *Neuron*. And triggering that reward center gives you a little thrill that stimulates and energizes you. It also keeps you coming back for more, increasing the likelihood that you'll continue incorporating new things into your life to keep feeling revitalized.

To counteract an energy dip during your day, switch to a new task or change your environment by going for a quick walk (even if it's just to the kitchen or a coworker's cubicle to chat for a minute). Getting up from your chair has another advantage: Movement can get your blood flowing and increase energy all by itself (▶86). Put a new spin on old habits by making creative adjustments: Handwrite a note instead of sending an email, order an unfamiliar dish at your favorite restaurant, rearrange a few pieces of furniture, or navigate your usual exercise route in reverse. For a bigger jolt of energy, pack several small new things into your day or tackle larger changes such as trying a new volunteer activity, learning a skill to earn a promotion or find a different job, or pursuing a budding friendship.

Banish Boredom to Reinvigorate Your Life

Monotony is an energy killer. In fact, a 2005 study in the *Journal of Sleep Research* found that monotony increases fatigue and, as a result, the time it takes you to complete a job, effectively prolonging the agony. While you can't avoid dull responsibilities entirely, you can make even tedious tasks less tiring by injecting elements of fun into them. Household chores, repetitive work assignments, sitting in traffic, and even waiting on hold during a customer service call can feel like they're taking years off your life. Not only does drudgery make you feel sluggish, it can affect your performance more than you may think. In a 2009 study in the journal *Accident Analysis and Prevention*, volunteers driving along a monotonous stretch of road rated their vigilance, or level of attention, as slightly improving over time even though objective measures of reaction time, brain waves, and heart rate indicated a steady decline. But finding creative ways to make unappealing circumstances more enjoyable can give you an unexpected charge, helping you stay alert, engaged, and full of youthful energy.

For example, do your most dreaded chores while talking on the phone to your best friend. If you have a competitive nature, make a game out of work tasks or turn them into a contest with a coworker. Create an upbeat playlist or download a new podcast to listen to on your commute, or embrace your inner kid and play the alphabet game, where you find successive letters of the alphabet on license plates, signs, and other passing objects (if you're playing alone, try to beat your best time). Treat yourself to a favorite magazine or a back rub while waiting at the airport. Seeing even the mundane parts of life as opportunities for fun or reward—a characteristic of the young at heart—can keep them from dragging you down and reenergize you.

The Takeaway: Rut Busters

In your free time, do something you've never done before. Visit a museum or a park on the other side of town, or have lunch with a friend at a new restaurant.

Vary your routine for novelty's sake. For example, take a different route to the grocery store—or better yet, find a new (and less expensive) grocery store.

Beat boredom by adding an interesting twist to mundane chores or monotonous tasks. Listen to music or a podcast, or wear something bright and cheerful.

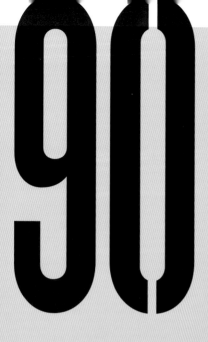

90

Restore Flagging Energy by Finding New Purpose

Learning, challenge, and motivation are all closely linked and can hugely influence whether you feel energized or bored and fatigued. They also help keep you sharp as you get older by forming new neurons and improving brain cell communication (▶33). And whether you start with a small goal or are looking to redefine the second half of your life, pushing yourself to aim higher can fill your days with meaning and revitalize you.

Set a Goal and Feel Young Again
Motivation is one of the three major components of mental energy, according to a 2006 study in the journal *Nutrition Reviews*. The motivation you get from setting and reaching a goal (so satisfying!) can invigorate you long after you've accomplished your objective, but the trick is finding one that will energize you and not seem like one more thing to cross off your to-do list. To get

inspired, choose a goal that's related to something you already enjoy. Planning for and anticipating your target may help you look forward to your favorite activities even more. For example, if you love to travel, start saving and making arrangements for a trip. If you enjoy making things with your hands, whether it's knitted socks or furniture, plan a few special pieces to give as birthday or holiday gifts. Compulsive journalers or letter writers might join a writing group and try to get an essay published or start writing a memoir.

Choosing goals with a social component can also help you maintain a strong network of supportive relationships, which protects you against energy-draining depression as you get older (▶30). If you can't wait for your weekly tennis game, set up a neighborhood tournament to raise money for a worthy

cause. Like cooking? Start a supper club or take a class to master a new technique.

Regardless of the goal you choose, expecting that you'll succeed can give you the energy you need to see it through, according to a 2009 study in the journal *Personality and Social Psychology Bulletin*. Setting high expectations can add extra motivation, and "hope can be a very powerful tool," notes Jason F. Mathers, Ph.D., a licensed psychologist in private practice. After your success, you might even be inspired to attempt a bigger challenge next time!

Age Gives You Perspective to Find Your Calling
All of the changes that come in mid- to late life, such as an empty nest, retirement, taking care of aging parents, chronic illness, or feeling burned out, can make you feel adrift and listless.

Adding purpose to your life can help you navigate these changes with energy to spare. J. Robert Clinton, Ph.D., a professor and author of several books about mentoring and leadership, argues that most people don't fully understand their calling—or see how their life fits into that calling—until they reach a stage he calls "convergence," which happens for many people around their fifties. It's not easy to get to convergence, he warns, but if you're willing to reach for it, all your past challenges and successes can come together to make this stage of life incredibly rewarding and invigorating.

To help you find purpose, ask yourself what your gifts, values, and passions are. Whom do you admire? How does this season fit into your larger life story? If you had unlimited time and money, what would you do to benefit others? Mulling over these questions can help clarify your calling and reenergize you to follow your heart.

Finding opportunities that line up with your core dreams and values can help you bound out of bed in the morning, eager to face the day. Experts agree that meaningful activities require both effort and using or developing your skills and talents. While work can give you a powerful sense of purpose, volunteering at something near to your heart or pursuing another passion can also bring fulfillment. Think creatively about how you might translate your interests into

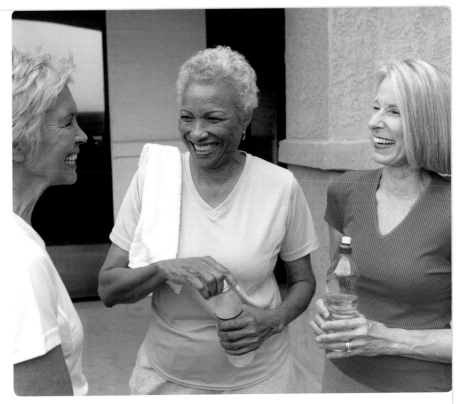

purpose-filled opportunities. For example, if you get fired up about gardening, offer to start a community garden in your neighborhood or at a local school, or teach a gardening class at a community center. Ask your friends and loved ones for their suggestions as well—the outside perspective can be helpful and encouraging.

The Takeaway: Finding Purpose

Set a goal related to something you enjoy: a craft, a class, a community contribution.

Consider your talents and expertise when determining your true calling, then seek out challenging opportunities that help you develop them.

Give back to gain fulfillment.

91

Boost Energy and Feel Younger with Aromatherapy

The interplay between mind and body, psychology and biology, can greatly affect your energy levels. And as your body gets less efficient at producing biological energy as you get older (thanks, in part, to increased free-radical attacks on mitochondria, the body's energy producers), mental stimulation becomes increasingly important to restore youthful vitality and keep your body active and energized. Integrative techniques like aromatherapy can increase your sense of well-being and send a cascade of reactions through your body that act physically to improve health and revitalize you. Although Western science hasn't determined precisely how it helps, accumulating evidence suggests that inhaled or topically applied essential oils enter the bloodstream and affect your emotional state with extremely few side effects, according to a 2006 study in the journal

CNS Drugs. So if you're looking for a safe, inexpensive way to counteract fading energy levels as you get older, give aromatherapy a try.

Centuries of traditional use indicate that aromatherapy can benefit your energy levels in two ways. First, it can relieve depression, anxiety, and stress, all of which sap energy and leave you lethargic (for instance, research shows older adults battling anxiety are more likely to report fatigue as well [▶85]). Second, certain scents are invigorating and immediately help you feel more alert. Don't fall for fake scents used in most air fresheners, candles, and personal care products, however. While you may enjoy the aroma, they don't offer the same biological benefits as essential oils. Look for products that list plant essential oils on the label, or buy unscented items and add your own oils. You can find

essential oils at natural foods stores; they generally cost between $5 and $15 for a 10-milliliter bottle.

Soothe Energy-Sapping Stress with Essential Oils

Research indicates the most popular scents to ease anxiety include lavender (*Lavandula angustifolia*), rose (*Rosa damascena*), orange (*Citrus sinensis*), bergamot (*Citrus aurantium*), lemon (*Citrus limon*), sandalwood (*Santalum album*), clary sage (*Salvia sclarea*), Roman chamomile (*Anthemis nobilis*), and rose-scented geranium (*Pelargonium spp.*). Which scent, or combination, you choose to help you de-stress and energize is largely a matter of personal preference.

Smelling lavender essential oil lowers cortisol levels and boosts your body's free-radical scavenging activity, protecting you from aging, according to a 2007 study in *Psychiatry Research*. Bergamot essential oil may also help minimize symptoms of stress-induced anxiety and mild mood disorders. Although researchers aren't sure exactly how it works, evidence suggests it acts on nerve tissue and protects the brain, notes a 2010 study in the journal *Fitoterapia*.

Some research indicates essential oils have an effect apart from their odor as well. A 2009 study in the journal *Natural Product Communications* tested topically applied rose oil on volunteers while blocking the odor with breathing masks. The researchers found that, compared to a placebo, the rose oil decreased breathing rate and blood pressure and increased the amount of oxygen available to body tissues, indicating that the oil subdued autonomic arousal, the body's subconscious control system. The rose oil group also rated themselves as more calm and relaxed than subjects in the placebo group.

Perk Up with Stimulating Scents

Research shows that peppermint (*Mentha piperita*), rosemary (*Rosmarinus officinalis*), jasmine (*Jasminum spp.*), and eucalyptus (*Eucalyptus globulus*) essential oils can erase fatigue. A 2008 study in the *International Journal of Neuroscience* noted that peppermint essential oil increases alertness and memory. University of Miami researchers demonstrated that rosemary essential oil gave volunteers a sense of relaxed alertness while lowering their anxiety

and improving their response time on math exercises. Jasmine increased autonomic arousal and alertness in a group of volunteers when applied topically, according to a 2010 study in *Natural Product Communications*. And volunteers who sniffed eucalyptus showed faster reaction times in a 2001 study in the journal *Chemical Senses*. Choose your favorite to offset flagging energy levels.

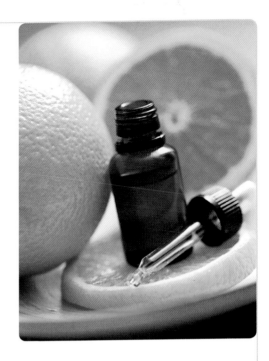

The Takeaway: Essential Oils

Sprinkle a few drops of essential oil onto the floor of your morning shower, or use products scented with them to get your day off to a great start.

Pop a peppermint when you hit a slump (scent and taste are closely linked).

Burn candles scented with pure essential oils to unwind and refresh after a long day.

Keep a bottle of your favorite oil nearby and take a whiff whenever you need a lift.

92

Bolster Your Social Support to Reverse Declining Energy Levels

Maintaining a strong social network as you get older offers a lot of benefits, from keeping your brain young and healthy (▶29) to keeping your heart in tip-top shape (▶57) and even supporting your immune system (▶64). Research shows it can also rev up your energy and keep you active and lively well into late life.

A 2010 study in the *American Journal of Industrial Medicine* found that airline workers who felt low social support were more likely to report symptoms of fatigue and difficulty concentrating. And midlife adults who expressed feelings of loneliness showed greater fatigue, low energy, and sleepiness in a 2010 study in the journal *Health Psychology*. Social support, on the other hand, can relieve stress and fatigue for middle-aged adults, note the authors of a 2010 study in the *Journal of the American*

Board of Family Medicine. Interestingly, whether the study subjects were married or employed didn't affect the results, indicating that having positive relationships apart from marriage or work has a strong influence on health.

Banish the Energy Vampires from Your Life

They drain your life force and can detract from the good relationships that will keep you healthy, happy, and energized as you get older. But even if you recognize that energy vampires need to go, it can be hard to pull the plug. So take a clear-eyed look at your history together to determine if you can salvage the bond by setting (and keeping!) limits, or if you're better off ending the relationship entirely. (Hint: If a connection continuously saps you, or if it compromises your values, it's not worth holding on to.)

Of course, you may not be able to cut off some relationships, such as those with family or coworkers, completely. In those situations, developing a set of coping skills to deal with the energy zappers can minimize their impact on you. Recognizing the real issues behind the symptoms of freeloading, complaining, patronizing, or whatever draining behavior is wearing you out can help you determine wise boundaries and perhaps even steer the relationship into more positive, life-giving territory. If nothing else, these associations are good opportunities to build patience, grace, and good conflict-resolution skills.

Mend Broken Fences for Better Relationships

Even the best relationships occasionally experience trouble, and that tension can tie you up in knots every time you think about it. Unresolved conflicts left to linger will drain you, as can dread about having to face the issue. But as hard as it may be to reach out, putting off phone calls, emails, or letters to settle the issue only prolongs the problem and eats away at you. To preserve your energy, and for the good of the relationship, you must stop procrastinating. If you need help figuring out what to say, ask a trusted friend for advice or write down your thoughts in advance.

If you're having trouble letting go of a grudge, however small, you might be interested to learn that unforgiveness can deplete your emotional energy and cause health problems over time, as noted in a 2007 study in the *Journal of Behavioral Medicine*. Other research indicates that unforgiveness leads to higher blood pressure and increased sadness, anger, and fear—exhausting emotions, to be sure. People who are able to forgive, however, report significantly more joy, pleasant relaxation, empathy, and perceived control. Maintaining a forgiving attitude might be even more important as you get older—young and middle-aged adults who frequently forgave themselves were more likely to report good health, but for older adults, being able to forgive others mattered more, according to a 2001 study in the *Journal of Adult Development*.

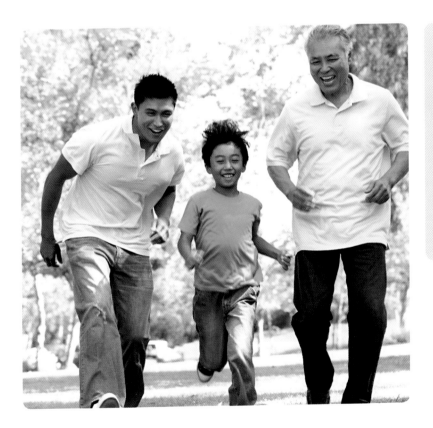

The Takeaway: Refine Your Relationships

Fill your life with rewarding social connections to help prevent energy-draining loneliness and depression.

Weed out the relationships that bleed you dry.

Repair energy leaks in connections you want to keep.

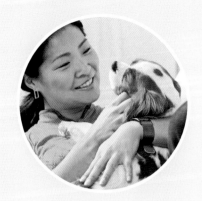
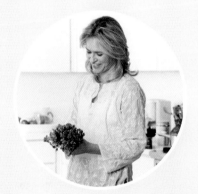
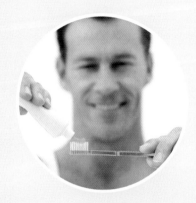
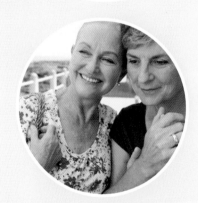
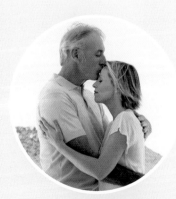
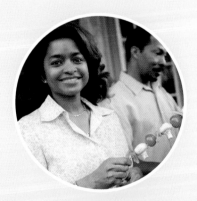

PART IX

Important Dos and Don'ts to Slow
the Aging Process

93

Don't Smoke to Live Longer, Better

Smoking is one of the biggest health threats we face today—not only does it shorten your life, but it can also steal quality of life in your later years. And studies continue to pour out describing the aging, harmful effects of secondhand smoke and even thirdhand smoke (toxic residues, including nicotine, that linger on fabric and other surfaces). Second- and thirdhand smoke can cause respiratory infections and chronic respiratory conditions such as asthma, cancer, heart disease, and sleep disorders, and it's especially dangerous for children.

It's never too late to quit and add healthy years to your life. Smokers who stop lighting up between ages thirty-five and thirty-nine live an average of six to nine years longer than they would if they continued, and quitting between ages sixty-five and sixty-nine can increase your life expectancy by one to four years, according to the American Heart Association.

There is no safe amount of smoking. If you need help quitting, talk to your doctor about resources and medications that can make it easier. Many workplaces and insurance companies also offer incentives. If you're not a smoker but are concerned about second- and thirdhand smoke where you work or live, contact your state representative to voice your concern or join an advocacy group (ask the tobacco coordinator at your county health department about effective local groups).

Quit Puffing to Keep Your Heart Young

Of the 440,000 deaths in America due to cigarette smoking each year, nearly one-third are due to related cardiovascular diseases. In fact, cigarette smokers are two to three times more likely to have heart disease than nonsmokers, according to the American Heart Association, and they're about 70 percent more likely to die from it. Smoking ages your heart by increasing your cholesterol, raising your blood pressure, and speeding up atherosclerosis—when artery linings thicken and fatty substances and plaque block blood flow. This increases your risk of heart attack, stroke, and other blood vessel problems.

But the damage can be undone—just twenty-four hours after quitting, your blood pressure and risk of heart attack decreases. Within one year, you'll cut your risk of heart disease in half, and after fifteen years, your risk will be as low as someone who has never smoked.

Long Live Your Lungs!

Your lungs have a natural defense system to protect them, but cigarette smoke interferes with that protection and leaves you vulnerable to infection and disease. Tobacco smoke can narrow your airways, making breathing more difficult, and cause chronic inflammation and swelling, eventually destroying lung cells and setting off changes that can grow into cancer. In a group of similarly aged volunteers, smokers' lungs appeared an average of ten years older than nonsmokers' (and five years older than past smokers'), according to a 2009 study by Japanese researchers. Smoking leads to breathing problems such as asthma, bronchitis, emphysema, and chronic obstructive pulmonary disease (COPD). And it's directly responsible for about 90 percent of deaths due to lung cancer, according to the American Lung Association. Ten years after quitting, however, your risk of dying from lung cancer is almost the same as someone who has never smoked. Quitting can also immediately improve your breathing and other smoking-related lung problems, including COPD, which is predicted to become the third leading cause of deaths worldwide by 2020.

Save Your Skin from Premature Aging

Not only does the repetitive motion of pursing your lips around a cigarette cause wrinkles around your mouth, but a 2007 study in the *Archives of Dermatology* found that smoking causes skin to age faster. The study's authors also noted that the more packs people smoked per day, the older-looking their skin was. Smoking breaks down collagen and inhibits your skin from making more, leading to inelasticity and wrinkling. It also causes blood vessels to shrink so your skin doesn't get as much oxygen; over time that hurts skin's ability to heal and leaves you with a not-so-lovely yellowish tone. Quit lighting up for good, however, and you can reduce these signs of aging, even if you've smoked for years. Secondhand smoke has similar effects, so avoid it as much as possible, too.

The Takeaway: Don't Smoke!

Tobacco smoke rapidly ages nearly every organ in your body, including your heart, lungs, skin, and brain, and it can even reduce bone mass and increase your risks for a broken bone.

Quitting now will add years to your life and better quality to your years.

94

Conquer Couch Potato Syndrome to Stay Fit for Life

Some research shows that, in terms of maintaining health and staying young, being sedentary is actually more harmful than being overweight, although they're often linked. For example, a 2005 study in the journal *Science* found that obese people sat on their duffs an average of two hours longer per day than lean individuals. But inactivity affects far more than your waistline. Prolonged sitting is also strongly associated with a decreased ability to process blood sugar, diabetes, metabolic syndrome, cardiovascular disease, and cancer, as well as overall risk of death, point out the authors of a 2010 editorial in the *British Journal of Sports Medicine*. Being sedentary for long stretches during the day puts you at risk for all those problems *even if you work out several times a week*. In fact, the study authors suggest redefining sedentary to mean periods of muscular inactivity rather than

the absence of exercise, so that people don't think they can go for a thirty-minute walk and then stay stationary the rest of the day. Both everyday movement and regular exercise are critical to keeping you young and healthy.

Increase Your Everyday Activity Levels to Stay Youthful

Older adults are generally less active than their younger counterparts, notes a 2006 study in the *American Journal of Physiology—Endocrinology and Metabolism*. But you can fight that natural tendency to slow down by intentionally finding ways to move more. Evidence suggests that even small movements—standing and stretching, going up the stairs to grab a coffee, or delivering a memo in person—to break up long periods of sitting is helpful.

If you find yourself glued to your computer, set an alarm to go off every forty-five minutes or so to remind you to get up and stretch your legs. Stuck in a car? You can safely stretch your arms and periodically contract and release your leg muscles or rotate your ankles to keep your blood flowing. If TV ties you to the couch, be warned: The more TV you watch, the higher your waist circumference, blood pressure, and other markers of heart and metabolic diseases (such as diabetes) are likely to be, according to a 2010 study in *Medicine and Science in Sports and Exercise*.

Exercise Smarter for Longer Life

Exercise can give you longer telomeres, the small pieces of DNA that protect the ends of your chromosomes and shrink with age. Scientists consider their length a good indicator of aging (regardless of how old the calendar says you are).

A sedentary lifestyle is linked to shorter telomeres in white blood cells and may accelerate the aging process, reports a 2008 study in the *Archives of Internal Medicine*. However, other studies show that exercise regulates the proteins that stabilize telomeres and keep them from degrading, while protecting against stress-related cell death. Aerobic exercise and strength training can also increase endurance, muscle strength, and balance, making it easier to be active in other areas of your life. (Research confirms that regular exercisers also move more in their leisure time.)

Experts recommend doing at least thirty minutes of moderate-intensity exercise on most or all days of the week. An even more effective approach might be interval training, or alternating periods of high effort with rest, which allows you to reap the benefits of exercise in less time. A 2008 study in *Applied Physiology, Nutrition, and Metabolism* found that high-intensity interval training (10 four-minute sprints separated by two minutes of rest) three days a week for six weeks improved fat burning, endurance, oxygen use, and strength. Research suggests it can also increase speed. Intense bursts of activity appear to enhance aerobic capacity, boost blood vessel function, build muscle, and lower blood sugar and improve insulin response more effectively than a workout of continuous moderate exercise, according to a 2008 study in *Circulation*. Because they're so challenging, intervals can also rev up a sluggish midlife metabolism longer postworkout than steady, lower-intensity exercise. Interval training can be strenuous, so ask your doctor if it's safe for you before trying it.

The Takeaway: Get Off the Couch

Limit your tube time to shows you really care about, and exercise while you watch.

If you work at a computer, get up and walk around for a few minutes once an hour.

Try interval training, with bursts of speed separated by moments of rest.

95

Don't Let Your BMI Creep Too High in Midlife

Researchers frequently use body mass index (BMI) to investigate how weight affects health. You can find a BMI calculator online, or you can measure it yourself by dividing your weight in kilograms by the square of your height in meters (kg/m^2). Overweight is defined as having a BMI between 25 and 30, while a BMI of 30 or higher translates to obesity (or being about 30 pounds [14 kg] overweight for a 5'4" woman).

Overwhelming evidence indicates that if you want to live longer—and in good health—keeping your weight in check is one of the most important steps you can take. When you're overweight, nearly every system in your body has to work harder to keep functioning, and the extra pounds throw your neuroendocrine system off balance: Fat cells produce hormones that raise your risk of type 2 diabetes, along with inflammatory substances that stiffen your arteries, heart, and other organs. In addition, excess weight can actually change your heart and blood vessel structure and function, and to meet increased metabolic needs, circulating blood volume, plasma volume, and cardiac output all increase. Thanks to those effects (and others), obesity ultimately increases your risk of stroke, cancer, heart disease, high blood pressure, sleep disorders, and type 2 diabetes over time.

Diabetes speeds up aging throughout your body and increases your risk of other unwelcome health problems, lowering your quality of life as you get older. Remarkably, diabetes diagnoses have doubled over the past thirty years, mostly in people with a BMI over 30. In fact, a large research effort called the Nurses' Health Study found that obesity was the most powerful predictor of diabetes—women with a BMI over 35 were nearly thirty-nine times more likely to develop diabetes than women with a BMI of less than 23, according to a 2010 report in the journal *Circulation*. All told, the researchers note, forty-year-olds who weigh too much shorten their life expectancy by more than three years.

Stay Slim As You Get Older

Maintaining a stable, healthy weight throughout midlife may benefit you even more than whether you're lean as an older adult. Researchers following more than 17,000 women for several decades found that those who gained the least amount of weight over the course of the study were not only more likely to live to age seventy, but also to be free of eleven major chronic illnesses (including heart disease, cancer, stroke, and Parkinson's disease) and have no substantial cognitive, physical, or mental limitations. And while being obese at age fifty increased their risk for health problems by 79 percent, what happened to the women's weight between ages eighteen and fifty mattered most, according to the 2009 study in the *British Medical Journal*. Those who had a BMI over 25 (considered overweight) at age eighteen and gained 22 pounds (10 kg) or more had the lowest odds of reaching seventy in good health.

So if you're under fifty and you've noticed the number on the scale creeping up year after year, put a stop to it now to improve your chances of living a long, healthy life. Of course, it's never too late to improve your well-being by slimming down if you're overweight.

Lose Weight to Live Longer

Lean people (with a BMI less than 25) cut their risk of premature death in half compared to those who are obese (a BMI over 30), according to a 2004 study in the *New England Journal of Medicine*. Accordingly, experts recommend keeping your BMI between 19 and 24. A 2010 study in the *Journals of Gerontology: Biological Sciences and Medical Sciences* found that a group of people who intentionally dropped about 10 pounds (4.8 kg) had half the number of deaths as the group who did not try to lose weight. See the tips in part II to help you slim down or maintain a healthy weight as you get older, or ask your doctor for suggestions.

The Takeaway: Lose Excess Weight and Keep It Off

Shedding even a few pounds can help restore a youthful figure, trim your medical bills, and add healthy years to your life.

Losing as little as 5 percent of your body weight can reduce your risk of chronic illness.

96

Avoid the Typical American Diet to Keep Your Body Young

Americans are big on snacks, sweets, and processed convenience foods, but as you get older and your metabolism slows, you need fewer calories to maintain your weight (▶12). That means there's less room in your diet for nonnutritious foods such as these, and you'll need to boost the quality of your meals and snacks to ensure you get the nutrients necessary for healthy aging while keeping your waistline in check. Processed and other "junk" foods cause problems because they frequently contain high levels of sodium (▶52), saturated and trans fats (▶34), and added sugars (▶55), which speed up aging throughout your body.

Excess sodium causes your body to retain fluid, leading to hypertension and making your heart work harder. Experts recommend limiting your daily sodium intake to 2,300 milligrams (1 teaspoon of table salt), but you'll likely find that eating processed or prepared foods takes you past that limit in no time. Looking for "low-sodium" on labels can help, but making your own meals using fresh ingredients gives you much greater control over sodium. As you get older, you'll benefit even more from laying off the salt: A 2001 study in the *Annals of Internal Medicine* found that people over forty-five who followed a low-sodium diet noticed a bigger blood pressure drop compared to their younger counterparts.

Saturated and trans fats increase inflammation that ages your brain, heart, immune system, and even your skin. You need some saturated fat, found in animal products such as meat and full-fat dairy, but experts advise keeping your intake to less than 7 percent of your daily calories. Trans fats, however, have no redeeming nutritional value, and you should shun them as much as possible. Pass on products that list shortening or partially hydrogenated oils anywhere in the ingredients list.

Added sugars, such as high-fructose corn syrup, are found in an astonishing array of packaged foods. They provide empty calories and send your blood sugar levels soaring, stimulating the production of advanced glycation end products (AGEs), which increase free radicals and inflammation. Continually spiking your blood sugar with sweets also triggers the release of extra insulin, which research shows turns off a "longevity gene" in your body. That blood sugar roller coaster also makes insulin less effective at clearing glucose from your bloodstream, accelerating the insulin resistance many people experience as they get older because of changing body composition (▶**21**), according to a 2010 study in the journal *Diabetes*. To keep your blood sugar steady, cut back on "white" foods such as flour and rice, eat more nonstarchy vegetables, and reduce added sugars to no more than 100 calories per day (about 6 teaspoons or 24 g) for women, or 150 calories or less per day (about 9 teaspoons or 36 g) for men.

Prepare Your Own Foods

The easiest way to avoid these aging substances is to cut back on processed foods and make your own meals. Styles of eating such as the Mediterranean diet (▶**13**) limit sodium, harmful fats, and sweets while emphasizing fresh, healthy foods such as fruits and vegetables, good fats, fish, nuts and seeds, and whole grains that offer an incredible array of age-fighting antioxidants and other nutrients essential to keeping you young and healthy. These foods are also generally free of preservatives, chemical

stabilizers, and artificial flavors and colors, all of which do you no health favors.

Another benefit of eating fresh, whole foods such as fruits, vegetables, and legumes is that you'll get more fiber, which helps you feel full on fewer calories and decreases your risk of diseases such as colon cancer, heart disease, diabetes, and obesity. Fiber from whole grains, in particular, is linked to lower weight, BMI, waist circumference, cholesterol, and blood sugar, according to a 2007 study in the *American Journal of Clinical Nutrition*. U.S. dietary guidelines recommend consuming three servings of whole grains per day. Good sources include whole-grain breakfast cereals, whole-grain bread (look for "whole-grain" at the top of the ingredients list), whole-wheat pasta, brown rice, popcorn, oats, quinoa, barley, wheat berries, and millet. Women should aim for 25 grams of total fiber a day and men for at least 30 grams.

The Takeaway: Your Live-Longer Diet

Limit sodium, sweets, and processed foods, especially those with trans fats and added sugars.

Follow the Mediterranean diet by eating more fresh fruits, vegetables, fish, nuts, and whole grains.

91

Steer Clear of Chronic Stress to Prevent Premature Aging

Chronic stress actually changes your brain structure, according to a 2007 study in *Physiological Reviews*, which may make it harder for your brain to "turn off" the stress response over time. That's worrisome because too much tension speeds up aging by increasing free-radical attacks, exposing your body to a continual flood of stress hormones such as cortisol, degrading your thymus gland and weakening your immune system, reducing cell communication, and creating constant low-grade inflammation, reports a 2009 study in the *Annals of the New York Academy of Sciences*. Overall, the researchers note, chronic stress leads to premature aging of key body systems that help you adapt to stress and respond to stressful challenges.

Continually high levels of cortisol can reduce bone density and trigger shifts in body composition as well, reducing muscle and encouraging fat to settle around your middle. That can put you at risk for osteoporosis, metabolic syndrome, and diabetes. Stress also accelerates some biomarkers of aging, including shrinking your telomeres, the protective caps on the ends of chromosomes. Telomeres naturally shorten every time a cell divides, and when they get short enough the cell dies, which may cause or contribute to some age-related diseases.

In addition to physical wear and tear, anxiety can also take a toll on your mental and emotional health. For instance, stress may make older adults more prone to depression, notes the American Association of Geriatric Psychiatry. It's linked to cognitive decline, and it can also drain your energy and keep you from appreciating life's pleasures. However, research suggests that lifestyle changes such as exercise, diet, and social support can actually reverse the brain changes brought on by chronic stress. That means managing stress can lengthen your life span while increasing your quality of life, allowing you to enjoy the healthy years to come.

Exercise to Tame Tension As You Age

It bears repeating that exercise is one of the best ways to beat stress. It can help you burn off extra physical and mental energy, boost feel-good neurotransmitters to lift your mood, and help you sleep better. It also directly counteracts some of the harmful effects of chronic stress that age you beyond your years, including strengthening your muscles and bones, keeping you trim, recharging your immune system, and warding off depression. In addition, exercise can actually slow the shrinking of your telomeres and protect them against stress-related cell death, according to a 2009 study in the journal *Circulation*. It also helps your body adapt to stress and be more resilient over time.

Interestingly, the stress response activates the reward center of the brain, along with the adrenals, the nervous system, and the pain relief areas. The reward is the relief you experience once the stress has passed. One reason why physical activity works so well to alleviate anxiety is because many people report the same thing with exercise— they may not enjoy doing it, but they feel so much better afterward that the promise of reward is enough to get them to lace up their sneakers.

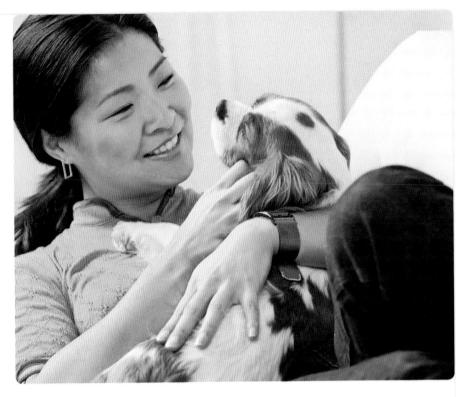

Change Your Perception of Stress to Slow Aging

You may not be able to eliminate chronic stressors, such as financial stress or caregiving, but you can change how you react to them. In addition to regular exercise and a healthy diet, sleep and good coping strategies are also critical. Restorative sleep can help refresh your perspective and make stressors seem easier to deal with. And healthy older adults practice acceptance, not worrying, and taking things one day at a time to cope with their stress, notes a 2001

study in the *Journal of Aging and Health*. Research also shows that maintaining strong social ties, pursuing religious and spiritual beliefs, managing your expectations and goals, and participating in activities you find meaningful can reduce stress and its harmful effects.

Additionally, you can teach yourself to elicit the relaxation response instead of staying constantly on edge. Try meditation, breathing exercises, yoga, biofeedback training, or even stroking a beloved pet. While doing these activities in the face of a stressor can help you calm down in the moment, practicing them regularly can retrain your parasympathetic nervous system (which helps you feel more relaxed) to be in charge more of the time.

The Takeaway: Nix Chronic Stress

Make sure you sleep well, eat a good diet, and get regular exercise.

Don't worry; change your perceptions of stressors by practicing acceptance and taking one day at a time.

Pursue social connections and spirituality to help buffer the harmful effects of stress.

98

Don't Forget to Floss to Preserve Your Health

One in three adults over age thirty and at least half of all noninstitutionalized people over fifty-five have severe gum disease, according to the American Academy of Periodontology. This serious bacterial infection increases your risk of losing your teeth and needing dentures. Not only can that make you look older than your years, but recent studies suggest that poor oral health, and particularly gum disease, can age your whole body. However, keeping your gums and teeth in tip-top shape can potentially protect you from heart disease, stroke, diabetes, cancer, and even cognitive decline as you get older.

Researchers aren't sure why or how oral health affects the rest of your body, but early evidence indicates the bacteria that cause gum disease also cause chronic inflammation. In addition, the bacteria buildup (or plaque) can enter

the bloodstream and release toxins throughout the body. People with high levels of plaque buildup are three to four times more likely to have potentially harmful bacteria enter the bloodstream after brushing their teeth or having a tooth pulled, according to a 2009 study in the *Journal of the American Dental Association*. The risk is even higher if your gums bleed during brushing (common with gingivitis and other gum disease).

A good deal of the research on the link between oral health and other conditions has focused on heart disease, and because of an increasingly clear connection, periodontal (gum) disease is now considered a risk factor. Whether poor oral health causes or accelerates heart disease or simply shows up at the same time is still up for debate, but several studies link gum disease to increased odds of having a heart attack.

Additionally, a 2007 study in the *Journal of Periodontology* found that patients with chronic severe gum disease had higher levels of the inflammatory marker C-reactive protein (▶49). Chronic inflammation ages your arteries and increases your chances of heart problems. Oral bacteria in the bloodstream also may lead to thickened arteries (a predictor of stroke and heart attack) and other heart conditions and contribute to the formation of blood clots. However, it's unclear if treating chronic gum infections such as gingivitis (the milder form of gum disease) and periodontitis (the more severe form) can reduce your risk of heart disease. A promising 2007 study in the *New England Journal of Medicine* found that intensively treating periodontitis improved patients' oral health and their blood vessel function, but more research is needed. Until we know more, experts agree it's smart to protect your smile—

and potentially your health—with good oral hygiene habits.

Keep Your Teeth and Gums Healthy for Life

A 2008 New York University study showed that daily brushing and flossing reduced the amount of gum disease–causing bacteria in the mouth after just two weeks. The American Dental Association (ADA) recommends brushing at least twice a day with fluoride toothpaste for two minutes at a time. Replace your toothbrush every three to four months, or sooner if the bristles start fraying. You should also floss at least once daily (if you have gum disease, your dentist may recommend flossing more frequently). If arthritis or other conditions make flossing difficult, ask your dentist about interdental cleaners that are easier to maneuver.

Other steps you can take include limiting sweets and avoiding all forms of tobacco. Bacteria thrive on carbohydrates, and eating sugary foods can speed up bacteria growth and dissolve tooth enamel. And smoking may be responsible for nearly 75 percent of periodontal diseases among adults, notes the ADA. But ten years after quitting, your risk of gum disease is the same as that of nonsmokers.

Overcome Challenges to Good Oral Health

You may need to put forth a little more effort to maintain a healthy smile as

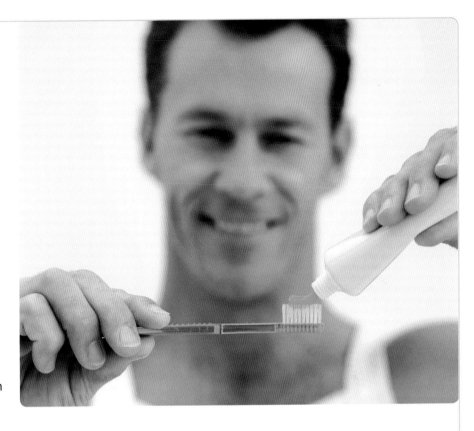

you get older because several age-related illnesses and conditions such as diabetes, stroke, cancer, heart disease, and menopause can aggravate oral health problems. Older adults are also more likely to take one or more of the several hundred prescription medications that have oral side effects such as dry mouth, which raises your risk of tooth decay and gum disease. Tell your dentist about all the prescription and over-the-counter drugs you're taking to help your dentist decide if you need to change your oral hygiene routine or come in for extra cleanings to maintain your pearly whites and protect your health.

The Takeaway: Healthy Mouth, Healthy Body

Brush twice a day for two minutes and floss once a day to prevent gum disease.

Limit sweets and avoid all forms of tobacco.

Conditions such as diabetes, stroke, cancer, heart disease, and menopause can aggravate oral problems, as can hundreds of medications. Ask your dentist if these are concerns for you.

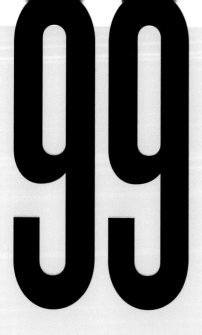

Don't Let Your Genes Shorten Your Life

When you think about anti-aging, your goal shouldn't be just to live a long life. You also want to embrace a concept called compression of morbidity, or delaying the onset of age-related illnesses and chronic conditions until very late in life to ensure you can enjoy and be active in your later years.

If you have a family history of heart disease, cancer, diabetes, Alzheimer's, or other conditions, your risk of getting those diseases increases. Likewise, if you have a close relative who lived healthfully to old age, your odds of doing the same go up. However, your genes don't tell the whole story. Certain lifestyle factors, such as diet and exercise, can change how you express those genes, influencing whether you develop certain diseases and how severe they are as you get older. In particular, researchers are investigating several "longevity" genes

that appear to affect your likelihood of living a long, healthy life. At this point, the best candidates seem to be genes that regulate inflammation, that are involved in the insulin signaling pathway, and that counteract oxidative stress.

Minimize "Inflamm-aging"

As you get older, natural levels of inflammatory substances increase, leaving you with chronic low-grade inflammation that scientists have dubbed "inflamm-aging." A 2006 study in the *Annals of the New York Academy of Sciences* noted that chronic inflammation promotes or exacerbates age-related conditions such as cardiovascular diseases, atherosclerosis, Alzheimer's disease, arthritis, muscle loss, and type 2 diabetes, among others. The researchers found that the increased inflammation by itself is not enough to trigger those diseases and to shorten

life. However, if you have a genetic predisposition to specific age-related diseases and also to strong inflammatory responses, chronic low-grade inflammation can cause real problems.

To keep inflamm-aging under control, eat an anti-inflammatory diet (▶25) and maintain a healthy weight as you get older (▶12). Body fat is hormonally active tissue, and it is one of the main sources of the inflammatory substances such as C-reactive protein and interleukin-6 that play a role in age-accelerating diseases such as atherosclerosis, insulin resistance, and diabetes.

Reduce Insulin Resistance to Halt Premature Aging

Insulin controls the processing, storage, and distribution of energy, and disruptions in its production or response can lead to obesity and diabetes, aging of body tissues, and possibly even cancer. Insulin resistance, or problems with insulin response and blood sugar metabolism, promotes oxidative stress and inflammation, both linked to premature aging, according to a 2010 study by Italian researchers. Animal studies suggest that altering genes involved in the insulin/insulin-like growth factor (IGF-1) signaling pathway can extend animal life span. (IGF-1 regulates cell growth and development, especially in nerve cells, and high levels are linked to cancer.) In humans, studies that have looked at centenarians found that they generally have preserved insulin responsiveness and low levels of IGF-1 in their blood.

Insulin resistance is more common as you get older, thanks in part to shifts in body composition to less muscle and more fat. But you can keep insulin functioning properly and slow aging by avoiding swings in blood sugar (▶ **55**, **96**) and building muscle through exercise—particularly strength training (▶ **21**).

Exercise also uses glucose for energy so less can build up in your system, and it helps your cells become more sensitive to insulin.

Fight Free Radicals to Live Longer

Genes that counteract oxidative stress, such as superoxide dismutase and paraxonase (PON1), may also help you live longer. PON1 activity decreases significantly during aging, while free-radical attacks generally multiply. Unstable free radicals steal electrons from nearby molecules, ravaging them and speeding up aging. Chronic oxidative stress contributes to age-related changes in immune function and other regulatory systems, such as the nervous and endocrine systems, as well as the communication between them, according to a 2009 study in *Current Pharmaceutical Design*. To decrease oxidative stress and lengthen your life span, the study's authors suggest getting an abundance of antioxidants through diet (▶ **26**, **54**, **67**). Brightly colored fruits

and vegetables (aim for five to nine servings per day), red wine, green and black tea, dark chocolate, and beans are all good sources.

The Takeaway: Go Beyond Genetics

Calm inflammation by maintaining a healthy weight and eating an anti-inflammatory diet.

Avoid spikes in blood sugar and exercise regularly to prevent insulin resistance.

Fight aging free radicals by consuming plenty of antioxidant-rich foods.

100

Don't Go It Alone As You Age

People with a strong social network live an average of 22 percent longer than those without one, according to a 2005 study in the *Journal of Epidemiology and Community Health* that followed nearly 1,500 people for ten years. Why are social ties so beneficial? For one thing, having close friendships protects against depression, which is increasingly common as you get older. That, in turn, may motivate you to take better care of yourself. Having a network of people you can turn to in times of stress or anxiety can also give you support and practical help, ultimately minimizing stress. Plus, loved ones watch your back and push you to see a doctor if you need to.

Social connection keeps you physically active as well. A 2009 study in the *Archives of Internal Medicine* found that older adults who were less social had a more rapid decline in motor function. The adults measured their social activeness on a scale of one to five, with one meaning they participated in social activities once a year, and five indicating near-daily participation. For every one-point drop in their scores, their physical function declined 33 percent (equivalent to being five years older than their actual age). If their scores dropped by a point in a single year, the resulting physical decline led to a 65 percent increased risk of disability and 40 percent increased chance of dying.

Note that studies show health benefits for a *strong* social network—not necessarily a *large* one. While having a diverse group of acquaintances, casual friends, close friends, and those who are like family (they might even be family) is beneficial, research suggests that those top two tiers are most important to your well-being. For example, while younger people may have larger overall social circles, both young and older adults tend to have the same number of close connections, which they agree is what helps them feel socially engaged. In fact, as relationships in the outer social circle dwindle, older adults may find themselves able to devote more time to close emotional ties and focus on those meaningful relationships. Having fewer than three very close relationships, however, is associated with loneliness, anxiety, and depression. If you've dipped below that, consider investing in other relationships to find another true friend or two.

Put Yourself Out There for the Long Haul

If your social circle is shrinking, you may need to make an extra effort to meet new people and stay engaged. Whether it's taking a class, volunteering, joining a jogging group, or attending a lecture at your local community center, there are countless opportunities to get involved and make new friends. Cast a wide social net, and be open to new places, people, and experiences. These things can be helpful for deepening existing relationships as well, and the combination of social activity and novelty can also help ward off cognitive decline (▶**29, 33**) and boost fading energy levels as you get older (▶**89**).

Pursue Faith for a More Meaningful Life

Being part of a faith community might also add years to your life—several studies have found that religious participation is linked to longevity. A 1999 study in the journal *Demography* found that white people who attended religious services at least once a week lived seven years longer than those who never attended—and blacks lived an impressive fourteen years longer.

The benefit partly stems from social connection and having a place to engage in leisure activities that are cognitively stimulating and encourage physical activity, notes a 2008 study in the *Journals of Gerontology: Psychological Sciences and Social Sciences*. Early research also suggests that religious men and women, regardless of race or ethnicity, tend to engage in healthier lifestyles. And a 2000 study in the *International Journal of Psychiatry in Medicine* found that

for women, attending religious services once a week protected their health just as much as avoiding cigarette smoking, doing regular physical activity, limiting alcohol consumption, and participating in nonreligious social involvement.

The Takeaway: Strengthen Your Social Connections

Regularly interact with friends and loved ones to live a long, healthy, and happy life.

Have at least three close relationships with friends or family members to protect against loneliness, anxiety, and depression. Nurture existing relationships while developing new ones.

Be part of a faith community to reap the benefits of social connections, physical activity, and spirituality.

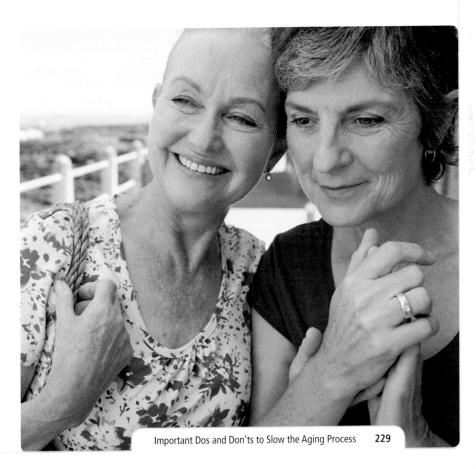

Acknowledgments

First, thanks to God, who opens doors I never dreamed possible. I also owe a great debt to my husband, Dan, who took on a multitude of extra responsibilities so I could write this book and who encouraged me every day. Mom and Dad, your support gave me the confidence to pursue a career in writing, and I am forever grateful. Cheers to my brother, Mike, who's also been bitten by the writing bug and shared in my excitement at this opportunity. A huge thank you to my writing mentors, especially Marjorie Stelmach, Jeff Seglin, and my former coworkers at *Natural Health* magazine—in particular, Daphna Cox. Your appreciation of language instilled a lifelong love of the written word, and your demand for excellence continues to inspire me.

Thanks also to John Gettings and Jill Alexander at Fair Winds Press for making this book possible, and to Laura Smith, whose editing and encouragement helped make the book the best it could be.

About the Author

Julia Maranan is an award-winning health writer living in the Boston area with her husband, Dan, and their dog, Sam. Formerly an editor at *Natural Health* magazine, Julia has written hundreds of articles for publications such as *body + soul*, *Shape*, *Fit Pregnancy*, *Family Circle*, *Fitness*, the *Boston Globe Magazine*, and Dr. Andrew Weil's *Self Healing* newsletter. She has also appeared on "The Deborah Ray Show," a radio program about natural health. Visit Julia on the Web at www.juliamaranan.com.

Index

A

acne, moisturizers and, 15

acupuncture, bone and joint health, 112, 113

advanced glycation end products (AGEs), 220–221

aerobic exercise. *See* exercise

 aging process, slowing of

 exercise, 216–217

 genetic factors, 226–227

 nutrition, 220–223

 oral care, 224–225

 sex life, 186–187

 smoking cessation, 214–215

 social support system, 228–229

 weight loss and control, 218–219

air quality, immune system health, 160–161. *See also* breathing

alcoholic beverages

 blood pressure, 125

 bone and joint health, 93, 107

 brain health and function, 69, 85

 caloric content of, 48

 immune system, 161

 sex life, 183

 sleep, 149

alpha hydroxy acids (AHAs), face and skin care, 17, 27, 29

alpha-glucosidase inhibitors, heart health, 139

alphalinolenic acid (ALA), face and skin care, 18

Alzheimer's disease. *See* brain health and function

anger control, heart health, 132–133

anthocyanins, brain health and function, 68

antibiotics, avoiding unnecessary, 162–163

antidepressants, sex life and, 170–171, 191

antioxidants

 brain health and function, 66–67, 68, 88–89

 face and skin care, 18–19, 28–29

 heart health, 128

 immune system, 156–157

apnea, 53

ArginMax, 190–191

aromatherapy, energy levels and, 208–209

astragalus, immune system health, 158–159

at-home skin treatments, 28–29

B

balance

 improving with exercise, 60–61, 98–99

 sex life and, 175

beta-blockers, heart health, 139

beverages. *See* alcoholic beverages; caffeine; teas; water

biguanides, cautions about, 139

bisphenol A (BPA), brain health and function, 86–87

bisphosphonates, bone and joint health, 115

blood pressure control

 brain health and function, 72–73

 medication cautions, 138–139

 sex life, 169, 170–171

 without drugs, 124–125

blood sugar (glucose). *See also* diabetes

 brain health and function, 67, 73

 energy levels, 200–201, 202

 heart health, 118–119

 weight loss and, 47, 52–53

blueberries, brain function and, 68

body fat, tracking of, 62–63

body mass index (BMI)

 aging process, 218–219

 bone and joint health, 100

 heart health, 125

bone mineral density (BND) test, 92–93

bones and joints

 alternative therapies, 112–113

 diet and nutrition, 102–107

 flexibility and stability, 98–99

 glucosamine and chondroitin, 108–109